D0060311

THE
SLEEP
FIX

Practical, Proven, and Surprising
Solutions for Insomnia, Snoring,
Shift Work, and More

Diane Macedo

wm

WILLIAM MORROW

An Imprint of HarperCollinsPublishers

HarperCollins books may be purchased for educational, business, or sales promotional use. For information, please email the Special Markets Department at SPsales@harpercollins.com.

FIRST EDITION

Designed by Bonni Leon-Berman

Library of Congress Cataloging-in-Publication Data has been applied for.

ISBN 978-0-06-304002-1

21 22 23 24 25 LSC 10 9 8 7 6 5 4 3 2 1

This book is dedicated to my cousin,
Victor. I still miss you every day.

CONTENTS

Author's Note   ix

Introduction   1

PART 1: THE BASICS   9
1. Identifying the Problem   11
2. Insomnia 101   41

PART 2: SLEEP DRIVE VS. AROUSAL   55
3. Overactive Mind   59
4. Sleep Confidence and Misperception   77
5. Not Sleepy Enough   85

PART 3: CIRCADIAN RHYTHM VS. SCHEDULE   105
6. Chronotypes   109
7. Scheduling   115
8. Light/Dark Contrast   125
9. The Right Way to Take Melatonin   139
10. Body Temperature   145
11. Meal Timing   153
12. When to Work Out   161
13. Sleep Debt Strategies   165
14. The Graveyard Shift   171

PART 4: SLEEP HABITS   195
15. Booze and Snooze   197
16. The Truth About Screens   205
17. Caffeine All Wrong   215
18. To Eat or Not to Eat   225

19. Sleep Nutrition   229
20. Relaxation Tools   247
21. Rethinking the Bedtime Routine   257

PART 5: SLEEP ENVIRONMENT   265
22. Let There Be Dark   267
23. Room/Bed Temperature   277
24. Noise   287
25. Snoring/Sleep Apnea Solutions   295
26. Mattress/Pillow   305
27. Sharing   313
Epilogue   323

Acknowledgments   331
Notes   337
Index   357

AUTHOR'S NOTE

THIS BOOK IS not meant to be a substitute for professional sleep help. If you are already seeing a doctor or specialist about your sleep issues, please carry on and simply use this book as a supplement to that care. It will help you to, among other things, ask informed questions of those overseeing your care and may present some options they haven't mentioned or considered.

If you are not yet seeing a professional about your sleep issues, I hope the information in this book empowers you to finally address them. But it is important to consult with your doctor before trying any of the interventions in this book.

INTRODUCTION

FOR AS LONG as I can remember, sleep and I have had a complicated relationship. In fact, it started even before I can remember. My mom often recalls what a "terrible sleeper" I was as a baby. Every night I would wake up in a teething-related coughing fit and then stay awake for two hours before finally falling back asleep.

With so little sleep during the night, I should have slept all day. But nope. Mom says, "You were never a nap taker. You would sleep very little during the day. But you were a happy baby!"

This was a sharp contrast to my older sister and younger brother, who were always very "good sleepers." Still, Mom says she never worried about my sleep. With my good disposition and otherwise good health, she said it was pretty clear that I just didn't need as much sleep as they did.

That trend continued as I hit school age. When everyone else was having naptime, I was wide awake, wondering how much longer I would have to lie there. And Mom noticed something else about my sleep habits: given the choice, I always went to bed later than my siblings.

In high school and college, I considered my ability to stay up late an asset. It helped me cram for tests and write papers until the wee hours, and also served me well in my late-night jobs: waitressing, bartending, and singing. When I recently asked my college roommate, Amy, if I ever complained about being tired during those years, she answered, "Never! You were a machine." But when I started working early morning news hours, that machine started to break down.

My 3:00 A.M. wake-up call during my time at the Fox Business Network welcomed me to the world of acid reflux. When that wake-up time shifted to 1:30 A.M. at CBS New York, I was a mess. The problem was, I couldn't fall asleep before 10:00 or 11:00 P.M., no matter what time I went to bed. After only three and a half hours of sleep, I would feel awful all day. I'd spend the day longing to be back in bed. When I finally got home around 4:00 P.M., I couldn't fall asleep. After a while, even sleeping during "normal" hours became difficult. I would sometimes go days without sleeping, even when I didn't have to get up for work.

Finally I went to my doctor. She prescribed Ambien and convinced me to at least take it when I had a string of sleepless nights. I was very hesitant about taking a sleeping pill, but I was desperate, so I agreed to give it a try. Thus began another complicated relationship.

Ambien, to me, was a miracle drug. I would take half of this tiny pill, and like magic, in half an hour I would be asleep. Sun still up? Asleep. Super Bowl party in the next room? Asleep. Stuck in the world's least comfortable airplane seat? Asleep! But I would come to need that Ambien more and more once I moved to the overnight shift at ABC News.

Anchoring *World News Now* and *America This Morning* was probably the best job I'll ever have. But simply put, it broke me, and not for the reasons you might expect. Working 10:00 P.M. to 6:00 A.M. was surprisingly manageable. It felt like a really late night out, which we've already established I can do.

But when I started making regular appearances on *Good Morning America*, 6:00 A.M. became 9:00 A.M. Suddenly it wasn't so much a late night as it was legit sleeping during the day. And if I was bad at that as a baby, just imagine how terrible I am at it as an adult.

Sleeping when I got home became increasingly difficult, and any disruption to my sleep schedule—like a midday shoot—would completely throw me off. My already low five hours of daily sleep would drop to one or two hours, even though I was spending up to twelve hours in bed. Then it would take weeks to build back up to my usual five hours of sleep.

My trouble wasn't just falling asleep, it was also staying asleep. On a good day, I would wake up several times. On a bad day, I would wake up only once—because I was never able to fall back asleep.

Perhaps not coincidentally, this was all happening amid the beginning of a cultural attitude shift toward sleep. Arianna Huffington came out with her book *The Sleep Revolution*, and the conversation surrounding sleep started to change. Sleep was no longer an inconvenience or a sign of laziness; instead it was something to cherish, respect, even revere. Matthew Walker followed with his book *Why We Sleep*, and more and more the message was cemented: If you don't get the "recommended eight hours" of sleep a day—you're basically doomed.

The more I heard that message, the more I worried. I hadn't gotten eight hours a night in my entire adult life! But the harder I tried to sleep, the less sleep I got. Terrified of the damage I was doing to my body, I upped my occasional Ambien to twice a week.

On most days, everything hurt. I managed to keep it together on TV, but behind the scenes my eyes felt dry and achy; I had permanent heartburn that seemed to radiate through my body; my mind felt foggy, slow, and impossible to focus; and I somehow also felt hyper, with racing thoughts and a racing heart. On my Ambien days, I got a bit more sleep and my physical state went from awful to bearable. I really looked forward to that twice-a-week "break."

And then one day, the magic stopped. I took my usual half an Ambien, got in bed, and . . . nothing. I couldn't fall asleep. I waited a week or two before trying Ambien again. Again, it made no difference. My doctor said that since I was on half of the lowest dosage, I could try taking a full pill, but the idea that I had developed a tolerance to sleeping pills—and maybe even a dependency on them—was a wake-up call. I knew in that moment this was not a viable long-term solution for me, and I was determined to find a better one.

I started reading a lot about sleep and trying lots of different remedies—from teas and oils to sleep hygiene and the "perfect," screen-free bedtime routine—but it all seemed to make my sleep worse.

I also found a lot of disheartening info. Essentially, if I wanted to sleep well, I would need to, among other things:

- Swear off unhealthy food
- Swear off alcohol
- Swear off caffeine
- Sleep in accordance with my circadian rhythm—aka, quit my job
- Sleep with my phone outside the bedroom—aka, find a new career, because working in news requires you to be reachable at all times

The thing is, I love my job, I love food, and drinking (in moderation) brings me pleasure. In order to sleep, I had to give all that up? Refuse and be doomed to lifelong sleep deprivation? I just couldn't accept that.

I'm a journalist. I'm into finding answers to difficult questions. I'm also a consummate DIYer and life hacker who loves analyzing problems and finding practical, nonobvious solutions. With the help of those skills and the guidance of a sleep specialist, I managed the seemingly impossible: despite being light-sensitive, sound-sensitive, temperature-sensitive, a light sleeper, a night owl, and having at least two different kinds of insomnia . . . I started getting a full night's sleep—in the middle of the day.

Since telling my story on *World News Now* and *Good Morning America,* I've been inundated with questions from viewers, friends, and colleagues seeking advice about their sleep troubles. It's now clear to me: anyone can have trouble sleeping—no matter what shift you work, no matter how rich and famous you are, and no matter how polished and perfect you might seem.

And while not everyone thinks their problems rise to the level of needing medical attention, there's plenty you can do right now at home, to help you get better sleep.

A lot has changed since I started on this journey—including a new work schedule, a new baby, and a new normal because of the Covid-19 pandemic. But one thing hasn't changed: I'm still satisfied with my sleep. That's not to say that every night is perfect. But now if I don't sleep enough, it's usually because I chose to do something else with my time—not because I couldn't sleep. And if I have a bad night, I know exactly what to do to get back on track.

My hope with this book is to pass that on to you, by giving you not only an array of tools that will work for you right now but also an understanding of *why* these things work. It's that understanding that has allowed me to continuously adjust these tools to navigate sleep in what continues to be an imperfect life.

It's better sleep, on my terms. I hope this book helps you get better sleep, on yours.

How to Use This Book

The Sleep Fix is best read chronologically, but if you choose to skip around, please read chapter 1 before you do, and use that as a guide for where to go next. This is important for two reasons:

1. It's easy to confuse different sleep issues that require different solutions, so you want to make sure you're using the right tools for your issue.
2. Some tools in this book, particularly toward the back of the book, are good for generally improving sleep but are largely ineffective against sleep disorders. Trying to use these tools before addressing the underlying issue that's keeping you awake will likely leave you frustrated—which, ironically, can aggravate or even cause insomnia. Trust me, I say this from experience.

If after reading chapter 1 you believe you have insomnia, then read through chapter 3 so you can learn about some of the lesser-known causes of insomnia—like conditioned arousal.

Then if you suspect you have conditioned arousal, read all of part 2 before moving on to any other parts of this book. Not only will these chapters help address your conditioned arousal—which is crucial to overcoming insomnia—but what you learn there can also help improve your chances of reaping the benefits of the rest of the tools in this book.

If the description of conditioned arousal doesn't sound familiar, that's an indication that your insomnia might still be in the early stages or insomnia is not the cause of your sleep problems. The rest of the book should help to shed some light on other potential causes and solutions.

It's also worth noting that this book is very comprehensive, with expert insights from many different areas of sleep science. I've tried to prioritize things in order of believed effectiveness to help you decide where to start, but remember: you don't have to do it all, you don't have to do it perfectly, and you don't have to do it forever.

My unscientific advice? To the extent it doesn't contradict the instructions above, pick whatever seems like the easiest and/or most effective change for you and go from there. For example, as someone who loves food and can't sleep on an empty stomach, I knew any sleep tool that involved restricting my eating was not going to be the best starting point for me. But simple strategies to improve my light exposure seemed very doable and I suspected they'd be especially effective given my overnight work schedule. I was right.

This is important because one of the things that can seem most daunting about sleep disorders is they often feed on themselves, creating more sleep obstacles along the way. It can feel like you're falling down a sleepless black hole with no way out. But just as sleep problems lead to more sleep problems, the process works in reverse, too. Sometimes finding just one place to start, one thread to pull on, can shift the momentum in the other direction—sleep improvement leads to more sleep improvement.

So let's get started.

PART 1

THE BASICS

Two main systems drive us to wake up and fall asleep every day: sleep drive and circadian rhythm.

- Sleep drive is like hunger. The longer we go without eating, the hungrier we feel. Similarly, the longer we go without sleeping, the higher our sleep drive—aka the sleepier we feel. Then, just as eating makes hunger go away, sleeping makes our sleep drive go away. When we wake up, the process starts all over again.

Sleep Drive

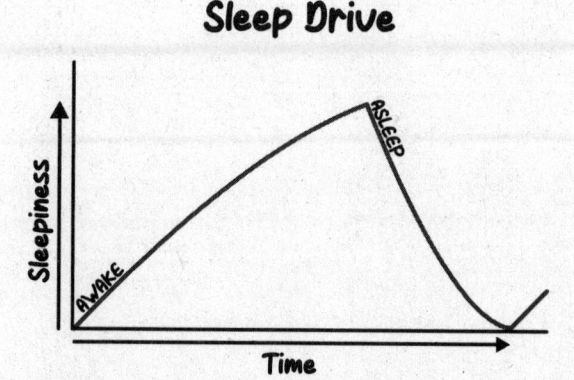

- Circadian rhythm, on the other hand, is like an internal clock that sends our body wake signals at certain times of the day—regardless of whether or not we've slept.

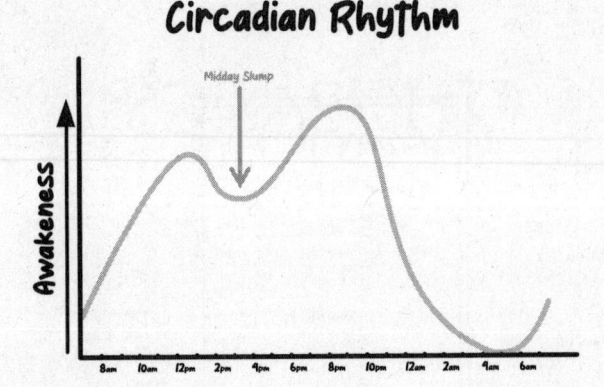

If you have issues sleeping, something is interfering with one or both of these systems.

The first step toward fixing your sleep is to figure out what.

CHAPTER 1

Identifying the Problem

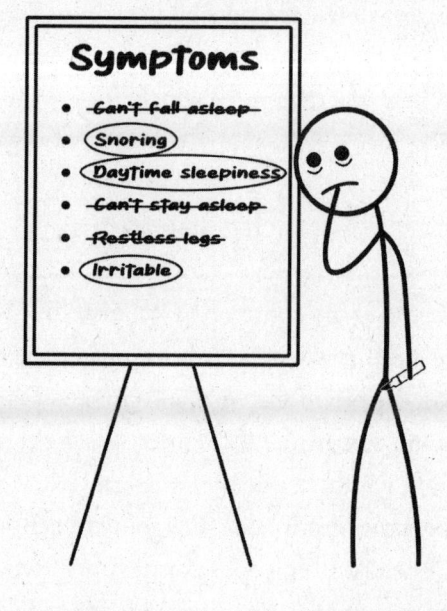

THERE'S NO POINT IN TRYING a bunch of solutions for a sleep problem you don't have. But you'd be surprised how frequently people are treated for the wrong thing or aren't treated at all.

One reason this happens is that sleep disorders don't always present with their most well-known symptoms or red flags. Without the detailed knowledge of a sleep specialist, many patients—and sometimes their doctors—assume they have a different sleep disorder, a different problem entirely, or no problem.

People also tend to assume that if they're not sleeping well, they must have insomnia, and studies show that most people with insomnia don't seek professional help. That means a huge chunk of people are missing out on learning that their insomnia is treatable or that their problem's not actually insomnia.

It's also very possible to have more than one sleep issue. Treat only one of them and you'll still be left with a problem.

Of course, the best way to determine what's keeping you awake is to see a sleep specialist, but there are a few things you can do at home to narrow down the possibilities. This chapter aims to give you a quick summary of some of the more common sleep disorders and tools to help you determine which, if any, you might have.

Insomnia

Insomnia is the most common sleep disorder in the world, and arguably the most misunderstood. Even sleep experts can't seem to settle on one definition for what insomnia actually is. Sometimes it's a symptom, sometimes a disorder. Read three different books and you might get three different answers.

For the purpose of this book, I'm going to define insomnia as unexplained difficulty falling asleep or staying asleep, despite adequate opportunity to sleep, resulting in impairment.

Have you ever felt like crap because you couldn't fall asleep or stay asleep the night before for no apparent reason? Just couldn't stop . . . thinking? You have experienced insomnia.

The next question is for how long? If you just have the occasional bad night, that's completely normal and doesn't require any special interventions. But if you have insomnia on a regular basis, there are several steps you can take to address it.

Because insomnia is such a complicated beast, we're going to spend a lot more time in this book discussing why it happens and how to fix it. Still, even if you feel confident you have insomnia, be sure to read the rest of this chapter. Insomnia is especially easy to confuse with other sleep issues and frequently coexists with them. Let's ensure you're addressing the right problem and the *whole* problem.

Circadian Rhythm Disorders

Circadian rhythm disorders are a timing issue. They happen if we regularly try to sleep when our body naturally wants to be awake. But it can be tricky to differentiate a circadian rhythm disorder from insomnia because they present in the exact same way: you have trouble falling asleep or staying asleep, with no symptoms to indicate anything else is wrong.

In fact, even doctors can confuse the two conditions. A 2017 study led by Dr. Steven Lockley at Harvard Medical School found 10 to 22 percent of patients diagnosed with chronic insomnia actually had a circadian rhythm disorder.

This is also another area where the definition of insomnia gets muddied. Some sleep experts consider a circadian rhythm disorder to be a type of insomnia. Others tell me it's a separate condition. For clarity and ease I'm going with the latter group because the two problems have different causes and different solutions.

The easiest way to tell the difference between a circadian rhythm disorder and insomnia is that those struggling with a circadian rhythm disorder can get a good night's sleep when they're able to do it on their schedule. For example, if you struggle to fall asleep and wake up during the workweek but sleep fine when allowed to stay up late and sleep in on weekends, it's likely your circadian rhythm that's causing your sleep issues, not insomnia.

Luckily, as with insomnia, there's a lot you can do at home to troubleshoot circadian rhythm issues—some as simple as wearing sunglasses at the right time. If you suspect this is your issue, be sure to check out part 3 of this book.

Still, it is very possible to have both circadian rhythm issues and insomnia, like I did. In this case, you will need to resolve both. Parts 2 and 3 of this book should be a big help.

Sleep Apnea/Sleep Disordered Breathing

Sleep apnea is another common sleep disorder that's generally not taken seriously enough. It should really be called "sleep suffocation" because that's basically what's happening. Those who suffer from it repeatedly stop breathing in their sleep for at least ten seconds at a time—up to a hundred times per hour! Imagine someone was smothering you with a pillow or choking you over and over again all night long while you tried to sleep—you'd probably make it a top priority to remedy that problem ASAP. But while the body does wake up from an apnea to breathe again, those awakenings are usually so brief you don't remember them. So despite the severity of the condition, many sleep apnea patients don't even realize they have it.

For my dad, it wasn't until my mom pushed him to get a sleep study that he finally got diagnosed with sleep apnea. But Dad says in retrospect there were warning signs. "I thought I slept all night . . . but I felt tired," he tells me. Throughout the day, during moments of stillness, Dad would even feel the strong urge to nod off. "I would get involved with doing something else to distract my body, so I would not fall asleep," he says.

Dad now calls his CPAP machine a "godsend," saying as soon as he started using it, he felt "great." He explains, "[It's like] when you take medication for your headache and then the headache goes away."

Since Dad started treating his sleep apnea, his boost in energy and mood is obvious to anyone around him, and I couldn't be happier for him and for us. But he does have a heart condition and high blood pressure, which led to a nearly fatal stroke last year, and I wonder how much of that is due to the decades he likely spent with untreated sleep apnea. Because those breathing interruptions don't just disrupt your sleep, they also cause sudden drops in blood oxygen levels. According to the Mayo Clinic, these leave you at higher risk for high blood pressure, recurrent heart attack, stroke, and even sudden death from an irregular heartbeat. Sleep apnea can also put you at higher risk for type 2 diabetes, metabolic syndrome, liver problems, and of course car crashes and workplace accidents.

Adam Amdur, chairperson of the American Sleep Apnea Association, says he believes the heart condition and early-onset dementia that killed his father were due to sleep apnea. "My father had triple bypass at thirty-eight. I was six months old," he tells me.

Adam also had his own issues but could never seem to pinpoint why. "I was always a smart kid who got an A in calculus [tests] but a C in the class because I was too tired to do my homework. I started and stopped so many different film projects . . . I literally fell asleep at the wheel when I was twenty-seven years old in Miami with my best friend in the car—drove through a gas station," he says.

After the crash Adam went to doctor after doctor trying to figure out what was wrong. "They just said you're young and dumb. They assumed that I was doing drugs or I was drinking," he says.

Then years later Adam's best friend, Brian, had just finished med school and joined Adam and his family on vacation. Adam explains, "He saw me nod off in a chair in the afternoon . . . then that night heard me snoring through the walls. The next morning, he looks right up at my mother, through me, says, 'I know what's wrong with Adam, and Mrs. Amdur, I know what was wrong with your husband.'"

At Brian's urging, Adam went for a sleep study immediately upon returning home. He says within twenty minutes of being asleep, the tech paused the study and immediately started him on a CPAP machine, the first-line treatment for sleep apnea.

Adam says he woke up at 5:36 the next morning feeling like he'd been "shot out of cannon." "I was thirty-five years old at the time, and my brain felt like it was ten years old. I hadn't felt that fresh and that energetic and that clear in over twenty-five years," he says.

But Adam didn't stop there. Noticing warning signs in other members of his family, he pushed his mother to get tested for sleep apnea and even took his two-year-old daughter to get evaluated. Both came back positive. "I then realized not only that this was my life's problem, this ran in my family," Adam says, "and it was time to reach out and help others."

Both my dad and the Amdurs have what's called obstructive sleep apnea, the more common form of the condition. This is when the airway is blocked during sleep, usually between snoring. But contrary to popular belief, not everyone who snores has sleep apnea—and not everyone who has sleep apnea snores. In fact, the rarer type, central sleep apnea, has nothing to do with the airway at all. It happens because the brain fails to send a signal to the body to breathe, usually due to a severe underlying condition like heart failure. Central sleep apnea is harder to flag than obstructive sleep apnea, but thankfully, it's also extremely rare, estimated to affect less than 1 percent of the general population.

Obstructive sleep apnea, on the other hand, is estimated to affect 33 percent of U.S. adults between thirty and sixty-nine years old. It's even more common in advanced age. And many of those people are going untreated. For some, it's because they're avoiding the treatment, not realizing how many options are actually available. For others, as explained above, it's because they have no idea they even have sleep apnea. The latter is especially true for four groups: insomniacs, racial and ethnic minorities, women, and children.

Sleep Apnea and Insomnia

While sleep apnea and insomnia are completely different conditions, science is showing they may be more linked than previously thought. Several studies now indicate a large majority of insomniacs—up to 99 percent!—who wake in the middle of the night are unknowingly being woken up by sleep apnea or other sleep disordered breathing. Unlike standard sleep apnea patients, who don't realize they're briefly waking up, those with insomnia are sent into a state of arousal (not that kind of arousal) and have trouble falling back asleep. These patients often complain about waking to go to the bathroom, racing thoughts, anxiety, fatigue, but most don't complain about respiratory issues. So their sleep disordered breathing goes untested, undiagnosed, and untreated. They might even use sleeping pills to treat their insomnia, not realizing the pills can make their sleep disordered breathing worse.

Minorities and Sleep Apnea

While sleep disorders affect people of all races and ethnicities, according to the Sleep Foundation "there are strong indications that they have a disproportionate impact on racial and ethnic minorities." Sleep apnea, for example, "was found to be noticeably more common and more severe in Black people and particularly for Black young adults." And while this area is understudied, the data that is available shows a higher prevalence of sleep apnea among Hispanics and Native Americans compared to white Americans.

Studies have also shown that racial and ethnic minorities "have a high rate of undiagnosed and therefore untreated sleep apnea." So racial and ethnic minorities may not only be more likely to *have* sleep apnea but they're also less likely to *know* they have it and thus less likely to get treatment.

Women and Sleep Apnea

Women with sleep apnea are also particularly susceptible to being undiagnosed or misdiagnosed. One big reason is the myth that sleep apnea happens only in older overweight men. "That's the biggest misconception," Dr. Jordan Stern tells me, "not only in the general public, but it's a common misconception, among healthcare providers." Stern, the founder of the BlueSleep Snoring and Sleep Apnea Center, says that misconception is so strong he's even had patients come to him saying their primary care physicians outright refused their request to be tested for sleep apnea—solely because they were young, thin, female, or a combination of the three.

He recalls one sixty-six-year-old woman who had suffered a stroke and read she had a high chance of having a second stroke if she had untreated sleep apnea. Despite her concerns, she was not able to get her neurologist to refer her for a sleep study. So she sought Stern out on her own and asked to be tested anyway. The results showed she had severe sleep apnea.

According to the Alaska Sleep Clinic, women also often present with milder symptoms like lighter snoring and shorter apneas, and men are also less likely to notice their partner's sleep habits (sigh). So if your partner is a man, he's less likely to flag that you're having breathing problems in your sleep. Perhaps not unrelated, studies have also shown that women with apnea present with different symptoms. While men report snoring, witnessed breathing pauses at night, and excessive daytime sleepiness, women often present with symptoms like fatigue, difficulty sleeping, headaches, restless legs, anxiety, and depression. These symptoms are more easily attributed to other causes and are thus less likely to result in a sleep study.

It's also worth noting that sleep apnea becomes more likely during pregnancy and after menopause. So while there are other reasons these issues could impact your sleep, add sleep disordered breathing to your list of things to check. You may be tossing and turning unnecessarily.

Children and Sleep Apnea

Perhaps the most unfortunate group of undiagnosed sleep apnea patients is children. According to a 2019 study in *The Journal of the American Osteopathic Association*, up to 15 percent of children have some kind of sleep disordered breathing. Of that group, 90 percent go undiagnosed. These kids are often instead diagnosed with psychological or behavioral issues like ADHD. What they're actually suffering from is chronic sleep deprivation! This is extra sad because treating children is often as simple as removing their tonsils and adenoids. If that doesn't work, an orthodontic expander usually does the trick. Yet so many kids continue to suffer during such critical developmental years.

I had never heard of sleep apnea before my father was diagnosed roughly ten years ago, and I didn't know children could have it until my cousin Rosa told me what happened to her then-five-year-old son, Marco. "He started snoring loudly for his age. He could sleep ten hours straight, but he was always tired. And he had no appetite. All he would eat was cereal and soup!" she said.

This wasn't hard to believe. The kid was really thin. But what I didn't know was he was also constantly sick with ear and throat infections and being prescribed stronger and stronger antibiotics to resolve them.

Things finally hit a breaking point the day Rosa got a call from Marco's school nurse at 10:00 A.M. telling her he was incapable of staying awake. Rosa says he'd slept ten hours straight the night before. When she arrived at the school to pick him up, he fell asleep in her lap. Marco was still asleep when they arrived at the pediatrician's office; he couldn't even stand. The doctor diagnosed him with yet another throat and ear infection but found it odd he had no fever.

"I remember when I got home, I gave him the antibiotics. He ate soup and went right back to sleep," Rosa said. "But I noticed at times it seemed like he wasn't breathing, so much so that I woke him up, afraid that he would suffocate." Rosa told the doctor, who sent them to a sleep specialist, who ordered an overnight sleep study and—a year and a half after his problems started—Marco was finally diagnosed with sleep apnea. Shortly after that, he had his tonsils removed and in the same operation, had tubes placed in his ears.

When I checked in with her recently, Rosa happily relayed that Marco, now twelve, never had health problems again. "He eats everything, he always has an appetite. He sleeps normally. His grades even shot up—the teachers say he's like a different student!"

Marco's story has a happy ending, but it's sad to think he struggled for a year and half, taking powerful antibiotics unnecessarily. And in many ways he's lucky. His loud snoring allowed his mother to eventually flag the pauses in his breathing.

For some kids, the symptoms might be more subtle, like Adam Amdur's daughter. "She was showing some behavioral issues, and she had napkin psoriasis. We kept going to the pediatric dermatologist, who kept giving us the steroids, the cream, and something wasn't making sense," he says. His daughter also looks like him, which Adam knew meant she had a higher chance of inheriting his sleep apnea since it's often caused by facial structure.

Adam says as soon as he brought his daughter into the sleep clinic, the doctor said, "The apple doesn't fall far from the tree!" and immediately told Adam she had sleep disordered breathing, adding, "The study's just going to confirm to what *degree* she has it."

So when it comes to sleep apnea in kids, the American Osteopathic Association advises looking out for "restless sleep, excessive sleepiness, teeth grinding and jaw clenching, migraines, bedwetting, and irritability" and that children with tongue-tie, trouble latching, or speech delay might be at higher risk.

But I Don't Want to Sleep Like Darth Vader

There's also a fifth group going untreated for sleep apnea: those of you avoiding the sleep doctor because you don't want to spend a night in a lab or sleep with a CPAP on your face. I'm happy to report, you might not have to do either.

Home sleep studies aren't great at detecting all sleep disorders, but they have been shown to be very reliable in the diagnosis of sleep apnea. In fact, when sleep apnea is strongly suspected, Dr. Stern feels that home studies are actually preferable to a lab, because they're more comfortable, cost-effective, and accessible for the patient. He adds that for a lab study, "the wait list in big cities or very rural states could be up to a year, which is completely ridiculous because we can ship a home sleep test today."

As for remedies, a continuous positive airway pressure (CPAP) device, which blows air into the patient's airway during sleep, is considered the gold standard treatment for sleep apnea. But less than half of patients are estimated to consistently use their CPAP long term. This is why Stern often recommends alternatives like an oral appliance instead. As he puts it, "CPAPs are great, but they're not going to do the patient any good if the patient's not going to wear it." This is one of the reasons I enjoyed being his patient. He understood that being a good doctor isn't just about understanding science, it's also about understanding people, and realizing that the best solution in a lab might not be the best solution for every patient in real life.

Shaquille O'Neal, for example, says he is one of those 50 percent of patients who have a CPAP machine but don't use it. "It is just too loud . . . And then when I talked, I sounded like Bane," he says in an interview on dentalsleeppractice.com. Instead he just let his apnea go untreated. Then one day Shaq got an Instagram message from Dr. Jonathan Greenburg urging him to try an oral appliance for sleep apnea. Shaq says he gave it a try and noticed that with the device in his mouth he sleeps uninterrupted instead of having to "use the bathroom 90 times," and wakes up full of energy and ready to work out. "I always had a four-pack, but now it's more like a 4.8," he says jokingly. More importantly, Shaq says, unlike his CPAP, he uses his oral appliance every night.

For my dad, the CPAP machine took a little getting used to. "It was uncomfortable for a little bit," he says, "But now I really don't mind at all. As a matter of fact, it's difficult for me to sleep without it."

In his TedX talk, sleep physician Dr. Barry Krakow also explains that patients with both sleep apnea and insomnia don't tolerate CPAP well but do better with similar devices that adjust airflow differently, like an Adaptive Servo-Ventilation (ASV) machine. This automatically adjusts its air pressure to suit the user's breathing needs instead of providing constant pressure like the CPAP.

So in addition to checking out the tools below, if you feel sleepy during the day and you're not sure why, push your doctor to send you for a sleep study—especially if you have a large neck, a small mouth, crowded teeth, or a small jaw. And if you're avoiding a potential sleep apnea diagnosis, know that there are options beyond sleep labs and CPAPs. A good specialist should be able to talk you through them so you can decide together what will work best for you. (See chapter 25 for more on snoring and sleep apnea solutions.)

Restless Legs Syndrome

Restless legs syndrome (RLS), also called Willis-Ekbom disease, is a condition that causes an uncontrollable urge to move your legs due to an uncomfortable sensation. It typically kicks in at night (no pun intended) and when you're sitting or lying still for an extended period of time, and it can sometimes affect the arms, head, or chest. My mother, who now suspects she has RLS, describes her symptoms as a discomfort in her leg. "I keep moving my leg from one position to the other to the next, and nothing alleviates that tension inside," she tells me.

RLS can be mistaken for insomnia because patients often report difficulty falling asleep. According to the National Sleep Foundation, it can also be misdiagnosed for other neurological, muscular, or orthopedic conditions, or even depression. In Mom's case, she has twice discussed her symptoms with her doctor, who both times ordered scans looking for potential blood clots. When the scans came back clean, the doctor sent her home with a diagnosis of "your leg is fine." I'm now urging her to see a sleep neurologist.

The good news is, while there's still a lot about RLS we don't know, researchers have found a very strong link between RLS and iron deficiency, and that treatment of the iron deficiency "markedly improved, if not eliminated, the RLS symptoms." Some studies also suggest magnesium can help reduce symptoms of restless leg syndrome. And sleep experts often recommend regular exercise (not too intense); a hot or cold bath before bed; a heating pad; gently stretching and massaging limbs; and/or occasional over-the-counter pain medications to help minimize symptoms.

For more chronic or severe cases, see a sleep neurologist as prescription medication can help. If symptoms are mild, you can also skip treatment altogether. I'm pretty sure I have RLS, but I've never bothered seeking a diagnosis or treatment because it doesn't affect my sleep. It's also worth noting that lack of sleep can make RLS symptoms worse, so any tool that otherwise improves your sleep can also help with RLS. Same for PLMD mentioned below.

If you do get treated, but after your symptoms subside, you're still unable to sleep, you may have developed insomnia in addition to the RLS and will need to address that separately.

Periodic Limb Movement Disorder

Periodic limb movement disorder (PLMD), often associated with RLS, causes your legs to jerk, twitch, or kick while you sleep. It can sometimes be mistaken for sleep maintenance insomnia, which is when you wake up throughout the night, but PLMD patients often report restless or unrefreshing sleep rather than actual awakenings. Many are also unaware of the movements unless told by a partner.

If you suspect you have PLMD, see a sleep specialist, neurologist, or ideally someone who's both. Some studies suggest magnesium can help reduce symptoms of periodic limb movement disorder just as with RLS.

Parasomnias

Parasomnias are sleep disorders that cause people to perform actions while they sleep, like sleepwalking or teeth grinding. As is true with PLMD, patients might report restless or unrefreshing sleep, but don't usually know they're active in their sleep unless they're told about it by someone else, they find evidence of it when they wake up, or they wake up while performing the action. My husband, for example, once woke up looking at his own reflection in a mirror (he's still freaked out). And a former colleague would occasionally wake up to find all of his kitchen cabinets were raided and he was covered in crumbs and food packaging.

For this group, even if you suspect you also have insomnia, Dr. Jason Ellis, director of the UK's Northumbria Centre for Sleep

Research, strongly advises that you see a sleep specialist and/or neurologist and avoid any interventions that affect your sleep schedule.

It's also worth noting that parasomnia can be induced by certain medications, including sleeping pills. If you think your overnight behavior may be tied to a new medication, tell your doctor immediately.

Narcolepsy

What if I told you you could have narcolepsy and have no idea? It might sound impossible, since you're probably picturing a movie character suddenly falling asleep in some bizarre and hilarious scenario. In reality, narcolepsy is much less funny and often much more subtle, which is why people can go years without being diagnosed. It's suspected many even go their whole lives.

For ABC News chief meteorologist Ginger Zee, it took four years, three car accidents, and an observant and persistent boyfriend before she finally learned she had narcolepsy. One reason: When a person suddenly falls unconscious, we don't generally assume they're asleep.

Like the two times Ginger thought she'd "passed out" while in the cooldown portion of the aerobics class she was teaching. "I was like, is something wrong with my heart? The last thing you think is that you're falling asleep," she tells me. But Ginger's heart was fine. So was everything else she'd had checked over the years. "Nobody could really put it together," she says.

Narcolepsy can also sometimes include lesser-known symptoms like cataplexy, a short-term paralysis often triggered by strong emotions; or sleep paralysis, which happens when you wake up but parts of your brain are still switching out of sleep mode. So for a few seconds or minutes you can't move or talk. Since you're still partially dreaming, you might also briefly hallucinate.

Ginger's sleep paralysis got especially bad after a man started stalking her and her colleagues at the Michigan news station WEYI. In real life, she and her colleagues would often spot the stalker standing there and staring at them as they ran errands near the station. But in Ginger's repeated nightmares, he got increasingly violent. "Eventually the nightmare progressed to the point that he had me back at my house . . . " she says, "He would forcefully sit on top of me, clasping my wrists with his strong hands, making them like handcuffs to the bed. I remember feeling almost awake, but I couldn't move."

Then the nightmare escalated again. This time the man was armed with a drill, and this time, Ginger says, she was no longer sleeping. "He would put the drill bit to my forehead, my chest, and my belly button, teasing me by revving the drill before quieting it and tapping it to a different part of my body. I couldn't move even though I was awake," she says. After a few minutes the man would disappear and Ginger would regain control of her body, but it would take a little longer for her to shake the feeling that all of it was real. "It felt like a wakeful hallucination," she says.

Perhaps the most misleading symptom of narcolepsy is trouble sleeping at night. While patients are excessively sleepy during the day, some find when they finally go to bed, their sleep is disrupted by insomnia, sleep apnea, or any of the other disorders listed above. It's easy to see how this could be super confusing.

The other thing that makes narcolepsy hard to flag is, while you might find it strange if you fell asleep on your dinner plate, you probably wouldn't think much of it if you dozed off while watching TV or sitting in a waiting room. But this is often what narcolepsy really looks like. Instead of assuming they have a sleep problem, narcoleptics and those around them often assume they're lazy. This is especially hard because they're usually teens or even younger when symptoms start. "I would fall asleep in class . . . so in my mind I was being a slacker," Ginger says. "It really sent me in a tailspin, and I think that's where my depression started."

But while it's bad enough that patients, teachers, and parents usually overlook narcolepsy as a possibility, doctors do too. Instead, researchers say these kids are diagnosed with things like epilepsy, behavioral disorders, psychosis, or depression, then prescribed medications that "can adversely affect" their quality of life.

For Ginger, after four years of symptoms, her new boyfriend noticed some strange patterns in her sleep and flagged that she might have a sleep disorder. So she insisted that her doctor send her for a sleep study. Before the study was even over, the technicians diagnosed her with narcolepsy.

Now, with the help of medication, Ginger not only appears on national television multiple times a day but is also constantly working on new stories and projects. And when she's not working, she's often working out, cooking, or running around with her playful family. Not the life you might picture for someone living with narcolepsy.

While managing the condition and the side effects of her medication hasn't always been easy, Ginger says the big takeaway from her experience is: if you think you're sleeping enough and still feel really sleepy during the day, "just get checked . . . it can change your life."

Mental Health

Sleep and mental health are very directly related. Mental health issues can cause sleep issues, and sleep issues can cause mental health issues. But while doctors typically treat only the mental health issue and assume the sleep will fall into place, studies now show that's often not the case. But treatment the other way around usually does work. As clinical psychologist Dr. Nick Wignall explains, "If you have both insomnia and depression, for instance, it's often a better idea to treat the insomnia first. Because it's a lot easier to treat the depression when you're sleeping better . . . same thing with anxiety."

So if you are experiencing sleep issues and mental health issues, seek treatment for both. Since many sleep specialists are also psychologists, you may even be able to do this by seeing just one provider.

Substances and Withdrawal Insomnia

While drugs, alcohol, and nicotine can all disrupt sleep, it may come as a bigger surprise that coming off them can too. Insomnia is a common symptom for people trying to quit any of these, which not only makes quitting harder but can also create the false impression that the booze, cigarettes, weed, or whatever else you're indulging in is helping your sleep.

For example, THC, the active ingredient in marijuana, can initially help you fall asleep faster, make sleep feel more restful, and potentially reduce nighttime awakenings. But with steady use, you develop a tolerance to those effects. Yet if you try to stop using it, you can get what's called rebound insomnia from the withdrawal. "This may not always be apparent to the user," Dr. Ryan Vandrey of Johns Hopkins University School of Medicine tells me.

Vandrey, who researches the behavioral pharmacology of cannabis, describes an as-yet-unpublished study he did where 99 out of 100 patients said the key reason they used cannabis was that they needed it to sleep. But he says when researchers monitored how they slept on cannabis, the patients "were past the clinical threshold of disturbed sleep on almost every metric" and there were architectural changes in their sleep. Without the cannabis, he says the patients' sleep initially got "substantially worse," but "with sustained abstinence, their sleep improved, beyond the point at which they were when they were using cannabis."

That's not to say that there are no scenarios where marijuana can be helpful. For example, if a doctor prescribes marijuana to help curb nausea from cancer treatment, that may indirectly prove very helpful to your sleep.

But if you are taking any substance—including traditional sleeping pills—for the sole purpose of improving your sleep, you should be doing so under the guidance of a sleep specialist. And if you're having trouble quitting a substance because of the impacts of withdrawal on your sleep, know that a sleep specialist can help. Some of the techniques in this book might as well.

Also, it's worth noting that nicotine makes you less sensitive to caffeine, so if you're quitting smoking, consider reducing your caffeine intake as well to avoid being overcaffeinated, or that too can interfere with your sleep.

THE UNIVERSAL FIX:
A SLEEP DIARY

Keeping a sleep diary or sleep log is often the first thing a sleep specialist will tell you to do, but it can prove incredibly valuable as a DIY sleep tool as well. In my case, I did not keep a sleep diary and later regretted it. I just didn't want to take the time to do it. Ironically, I now know it would have saved me a lot of time and guesswork. That said, becoming too focused on your sleep and the details related to it can create its own problems. So do your best to keep a relaxed attitude toward your sleep diary, and remember, nothing in it is meant to be exact.

As for what kind of sleep diary to use, in 2012 a group of scientists studied a variety of them and came up with the Consensus Sleep Diary, which includes a Core version with only questions deemed essential, and an expanded version that includes additional questions deemed optional.

Sleep Diary Apps

Arguably the easiest way to use the Consensus Sleep Diary is via the free app at Consensussleepdiary.com. It allows you to log your sleep from your computer or phone and lets you choose whether or not to track optional items like alcohol and caffeine consumption. It also automatically calculates things like your total sleep time and your sleep efficiency—yay, no math!

Another free digital sleep diary option is the CBT-i Coach app. Its sleep diary is more limited, but CBT-i Coach has the added function of using your sleep diary info to suggest the best bedtimes and wake times if you have insomnia and want to try sleep restriction (detailed in chapter 5). The CBT-i Coach app also offers a host of great sleep info. You'll find more on this app and others like it in the next chapter.

Physical Sleep Diary

If you prefer to put pen to paper, you can buy a sleep diary or make your own using the guide below. Consensusleepdiary.com also has printable templates of the Consensus Sleep Diary available for download. For a child-friendly sleep diary template, check out http://www.sleepforkids.org/pdf/SleepDiary.pdf. And shift workers, see chapter 14 or go to sleepfixbook.com for a sleep diary made especially for you.

How-To: DIY Consensus Sleep Diary

Answer the questions below every day, preferably within one hour of getting out of bed for the day. Remember to note the date somewhere on the page. All times should be rough estimates. Do not watch the clock. If you miss a day, leave the diary blank for that day and resume logging the following day, dating your entries accordingly.

1. What time did you get into bed?
2. What time did you try to go to sleep?
3. How long did it take you to fall asleep?
4. How many times did you wake up, not counting your final awakening?
5. In total, how long did these awakenings last?
6. What time was your final awakening?
7. How would you rate the quality of your sleep? Very poor, poor, fair, good, or very good?
8. Any additional comments or factors that may have impacted your sleep (for example, menstruation, changes in sleep environment, a new routine)?

Optional additional questions about your sleep and the previous day:

9. After your final awakening, how long did you spend in bed trying to sleep?
10. Did you wake up earlier than you planned? If yes, how much earlier?
11. What time did you get out of bed for the day?
12. In total, how long did you sleep?
13. How refreshed or rested did you feel when you woke up for the day? Not at all rested, slightly rested, somewhat rested, well rested, very well rested?
14. How many times did you nap or dose? In total, how long did you nap or dose?
15. How many drinks containing alcohol did you have? What time was your last drink?
16. How many caffeinated drinks (coffee, tea, soda, energy drinks) did you have? What time was your last drink?
17. Did you take any over-the-counter or prescription sleep medication(s) to help you sleep? If so, list medication(s), dose, and time taken.

(These questions are from the Consensus Sleep Diary credited to Carney et al., 2012, and have been reprinted with the authors' permission.)

Sleep diaries can seem daunting, but each log should take you no more than thirty seconds. As sleep psychologist Dr. Jason Ong tells me, "The whole point is we just want some estimate of what your patterns are and your perception of your sleep."

After a few days, you'll likely start noticing patterns in your diary that shed light on what's contributing to or causing your sleep problems. If those issues require professional help, your diary info can also help you more quickly identify what kind of a professional to speak to and can enable that professional to diagnose and treat you more quickly.

My friend Brad credits his sleep diary—or "sleep calendar," as he calls it—with helping to uncover that his sleep problems were partially caused by his circadian rhythm. "What was clear on the sleep calendar is that I couldn't sleep early in the night," he tells me.

Interestingly, keeping a sleep diary can also lead us to improve our sleep habits. We don't want to admit in writing that we spent an hour in bed scrolling through Instagram or stayed up until two A.M. watching *The Walking Dead*, so we stop doing it!

Brad says keeping a sleep diary even motivated him to work out more and drink less coffee. "Just by the fact of me writing it down, I was more likely to exercise for longer and more vigorously. And stay away from caffeine later on," he says.

After two weeks, if you still can't identify any issues that might be causing your sleep disruptions, consult a professional (more on how to find the right professional later in this chapter).

THE TEAMWORK FIX:
ASK YOUR PARTNER

We hate to admit it, but sometimes our partners know us better than we know ourselves. This is especially true when it comes to sleep. It's not unusual for a patient to fall asleep in the waiting room, then answer no when asked if they ever doze in public; or swear they're silent sleepers, when they actually snore like a chainsaw all night. Doctors often find these patients' partners paint a much more accurate picture.

So realize that it's common to have misperceptions about our own sleep, and ask the people closest to you if they have any observations to add to your sleep diary. Their answers may surprise you!

THE MOVIE STAR FIX:
RECORD VIDEO OF YOURSELF

It may feel a little odd, but taking video of yourself sleeping can provide you with all kinds of insights. I did this using a home security camera I already had. Since the room should be dark, anything with night recording will work well—including a baby monitor. Bonus if it records audio too. When you get a chance to scan the video(s), here are a few things you can look for:

- Do you snore, talk, kick, jerk, grind your teeth, or sleepwalk during the night?
- At any point does it sound like you stop breathing? For ten seconds or longer? (*Note:* This is easier to flag using an audio recording app like SnoreLab. More on that in the next Fix.)
- Did you get up during the night? How many times? For how long?
- Did an external factor disturb your sleep—like a sound, movement, or light?
- Is any part of your body restless before you fall asleep or during sleep?

Cross-check your findings with the conditions described above to see if anything sticks out. Not only can the video offer you new insights into what's causing your sleep issues, but it might also show you you're actually getting more sleep than you think! If nothing else, it can be another diagnostic tool for your doctor.

THE RADIO STAR FIX:
RECORD AUDIO OF YOURSELF

To supplement your video recording, or if video recording isn't an option, an audio recording can prove very insightful, especially if you suspect you might have sleep apnea.

On the recommendation of Dr. Jordan Stern, an ear, nose, and throat doctor and sleep specialist, I used the SnoreLab App for this. Despite its name, the app records and analyzes not just snoring but any audible sound in your room, and shows you a visual that makes it easy to flag anytime the audio level changed. It also allows you to input data points like whether you consumed alcohol that night, to see how they impact your sleep sounds. The app also suggests potential snoring remedies and lets you track their effectiveness.

While SnoreLab is not a substitute for a professional sleep study or diagnosis, according to its website, it can "be useful in recording evidence of apnea, such as periods where there is no audible breathing followed by a sudden gasp or choking sound. You may wish to activate Full Night Recording and scan through the recordings to identify suspicious events."

If you suspect sleep apnea, you can then take the recording to your doctor or sleep specialist to help them make a diagnosis and offer you the best solutions.

As fate would have it, the first time I used SnoreLab, my air conditioner broke and made some horrific sound all night long. So that particular recording was not helpful in assessing my sleep, but it did help the repairman diagnose my air conditioner!

SnoreLab is free but some features (like Full Night Recording) require a premium upgrade.

THE OLD SCHOOL FIX:
THE SPOON TEST

One of the easiest ways to see if you're sleep deprived is the spoon test, reportedly created by the late Dr. Nathaniel Kleitman, who was a sleep researcher at the University of Chicago. The test measures how long it takes you to fall asleep in the middle of the day.

For a modern version of the test, buy the SleepOnCue app and use its Custom Nap function. Set the total nap time to twenty minutes and the wake time for one minute after you fall asleep. Then lie down for a nap while holding the phone and give it a shake every time you hear the tone until you fall asleep. The phone will vibrate to wake you up one minute after you stop responding or after the twenty minutes are up. The app will then let you know how long you took to fall asleep (if at all). Compare that to the guidelines in step 4 below to see what that says about your sleep deprivation.

If you prefer the old school spoon method, all you need is a reasonably quiet and dark bedroom, a spoon, a metal tray, and a timer.

How-To: Spoon Test

The following test should be done during the day, ideally in the early afternoon.

1. Place a metal tray on the floor by the bed, in line with where your hand would be when you lie down to sleep.
2. Set a timer for twenty minutes. This will act as an alarm clock.
3. Lie down while comfortably holding a spoon above the tray and try to take a nap.
4. When you fall asleep, the spoon will drop and hit the tray, waking you up. Stop the timer and subtract the results from twenty to see how long it took you to fall asleep. Within five minutes indicates severe sleep deprivation, within ten minutes indicates moderate

(continued on next page)

sleep deprivation, and anything beyond fifteen usually indicates you're getting adequate sleep.

Note: Insomniacs who are not getting enough sleep might still be able to stay awake through this exercise due to their arousal. More on that later.

If the spoon test shows you're sleep-deprived, address what's causing that ASAP. If you're not sure what's causing it, use the other Fixes in this chapter to try to figure it out and consult a sleep specialist.

THE GETTING TO KNOW YOU FIX:
QUESTIONNAIRES

Sleepiness Questionnaire

There are several long and detailed questionnaires aimed at helping assess our sleep. But on its website, Harvard Medical School has one that seems to get the job done in just three questions:

- "Once you have caught up on your sleep during weekends or vacation, are you still likely to fall asleep when inactive?"
- "Do you feel rested in the morning but then tired throughout much of the day?"
- "Do you doze off at inappropriate times?"

If you answered yes to any of the above, the website suggests discussing your sleepiness with your primary care physician or sleep specialist. Despite how common and normal it might seem, regularly feeling sleepy during the day and dozing outside of normal sleep times (for example, while sitting in a waiting room) are usually signs of sleep deprivation and should be addressed as soon as possible.

Sleep Apnea Assessment

The STOP-Bang Questionnaire is widely used to quickly assess risk of obstructive sleep apnea. It's not foolproof and doesn't address central sleep apnea, but it can still prove very helpful and takes only seconds to complete.

You can take the assessment below or at stopbang.ca/osa/screening.php, where the results will be calculated for you.

How-To: STOP-Bang Questionnaire

Please answer yes or no to the questions below to help determine your risk level for obstructive sleep apnea:

1. SNORING: Do you snore loudly (loud enough to be heard through closed doors or your bed-partner elbows you for snoring at night)?
2. TIRED: Do you often feel tired, fatigued, or sleepy during the daytime (such as falling asleep while driving or talking to someone)?
3. OBSERVED: Has anyone observed you stop breathing or choke/gasp in your sleep?
4. PRESSURE: Do you have or are you being treated for high blood pressure?
5. BMI: Is your Body Mass Index more than 35 kg/m^2?
6. AGE: Are you more than 50 years old?
7. NECK SIZE (measured around Adams apple):

   - For male, is your shirt collar 17 inches/43 cm or larger?
   - For female, is your shirt collar 16 inches/41 cm or larger?

8. GENDER: Are you male?

Scoring Criteria for General Population:

- Low risk of OSA: Yes to up to two questions
- Intermediate risk of OSA: Yes to three or four questions
- High risk of OSA: Yes to five to eight questions, or Yes to at least two of questions 1–4 plus Yes to question 5, 7, or 8.

(Proprietary to University Health Network. www.stopbang.ca, Modified from: Chung F et al. Anesthesiology 2008; 108:812-21; Chung F et al. Br J Anaesth 2012, 108:768–75; Chung F et al. J Clin Sleep Med 2014;10:951-8.)

THE SNEAKY FIX:
THE GOTCHA ALARM

If you wake up at the same time every night, it's possible that your problem isn't with your sleep, but rather with your sleep environment. Dr. Jason Ellis suggests something I like to call the Gotcha Alarm to help you find out. Set your alarm for five minutes before your regular awakening time and just quietly observe what happens next. Does an outside light turn on? An air conditioner kick in? Noisy neighbor arrive home? I've even been woken up by my cable box turning on for a reboot (I'm very light sensitive)!

As mentioned above, you can also record video or audio overnight and check that time for any disturbance, or simply set the device to start recording a few minutes before the time in question.

If you do find your sleep is being disturbed by something in your environment, see part 5 for more on how to fix that.

THE PROFESSIONAL FIX:
FINDING THE RIGHT SLEEP SPECIALIST

If you decide it's time to get professional help, it's so important to find the RIGHT professional. Weekend *Good Morning America* anchor Whit Johnson says over the course of roughly twenty years he saw over half a dozen sleep specialists for his insomnia before finally finding one that helped him. "I kept getting referred to someone who was supposedly going to help me with my sleep, but at the end of the day was not a true sleep expert," he tells me.

But it's likely the people treating Whit actually were experts on sleep—they just weren't experts on insomnia. That's because sleep specialists often focus on a specific area of sleep, so you can be an expert on one sleep condition and know very little about another.

I made the same mistake. I met my sleep doctor, Jordan Stern, at a speaking event. He gave a presentation on sleep before a sit-down dinner, and I happened to be seated next to him. After talking to him all night, I asked him to treat me. I liked him and figured, *Well, he's a sleep expert, so he must be an expert on insomnia.* But while Stern is a legit medical sleep specialist, as an ear, nose, and throat doctor, his real specialty is sleep apnea. Insomnia and sleep apnea are two completely different conditions.

To be clear, Stern is an excellent doctor, and in the end I got where I needed to be. But if I knew then what I know now, I would have made sure to see a sleep specialist who specializes in insomnia. So if you're asking your primary care physician to recommend a specialist, be sure to ask about the specific areas of sleep that specialist focuses on. Here are some other great resources:

- Sleepeducation.org lets you search for sleep centers certified by the American Academy of Sleep Medicine (AASM).
- Behavioralsleep.org offers a directory of behavioral sleep medicine providers.
- Babysleep.com's "cool stuff" tab links to a search for AASM.
- Support groups for specific conditions can provide related referrals.

If you suspect you have insomnia, you'll want a provider qualified to administer cognitive behavioral therapy for insomnia or CBT-I. More on that in the next chapter.

Also, for those intimidated by the idea of an overnight sleep study, take comfort in knowing many sleep problems don't require one. As mentioned above, you can even be evaluated from home for sleep apnea. So don't be shy, reach out to a provider.

Dr. Christina Pierpaoli Parker, a sleep researcher at the University of Alabama at Birmingham, suggests once you do contact a professional, ask specific questions about the percentage of patients they've seen with your suspected condition, what kind of evidence-based assessments and treatments they use, what their remission rates are, and what training and certification they have. Also, ask if your health insurance will cover your treatment, and ask yourself how you feel about the provider. Having a good rapport can impact the success of your treatment.

Pierpaoli Parker adds, "Remain open to possibilities in terms of (alternative) diagnoses, treatments, and doctors."

CHAPTER 2

Insomnia 101

IF AFTER READING CHAPTER 1, you're pretty sure you have insomnia, welcome to the very large club. Despite its scary-sounding name, insomnia is incredibly common. Conservative estimates show anywhere from 10 to 30 percent of adults have chronic insomnia, and some studies put it as high as 60 percent!

But despite the prevalence of insomnia, it's amazing how little most people know about it. So before we start our deep dive, let's cover some basics.

Insomnia Is Not "Just How You Are"

I can't tell you how many times I've heard some variation of "I don't have insomnia, I just don't sleep" or "I'm a bad sleeper, that's just how I'm built." People tend to assume that either their constant difficulty sleeping doesn't "count" as insomnia or that insomnia is just a part of who they are, not a medical condition. This, as mentioned in chapter 1, leads most insomniacs to never seek treatment, despite the fact that insomnia *is* a condition, and a treatable one.

One of these people is my mother. "I was always a bad sleeper, since I was a girl," she tells me. I can remember while I was growing up how frequently she would complain about trouble sleeping and how often I would find her in the living room in the middle of the night reading or watching TV. (It definitely put a damper on my many attempts to sneak in late as a teenager!) Yet when I recently asked her if she's ever mentioned her sleep issues to any of her doctors, Mom said no.

This is especially interesting because it was my mother who pushed my father to get a sleep study after years of hearing him snore and hold his breath throughout the night. She tried to explain the difference to me, saying, "If I had Daddy's problem, I would address it, because Daddy wasn't sleeping." But then she seemed to have a lightbulb moment, adding after a long pause, "And I'm not sleeping, either." Still, unlike my dad's sleep apnea, which Mom viewed as a medical problem, like so many others, she saw insomnia as just "the way I am."

My friend Brad did the same. As a self-described lifelong insomniac, Brad says he'd given up on being a normal sleeper. "I've just always been operating from the point of view that I've dealt with this my whole life, I've always been able to function . . . I can survive, even if it sucks."

Then about a year ago, Brad's primary care physician retired. His new doctor asked Brad about his medical history, and specifically about his sleep. When Brad described his issues, the doctor referred him to a sleep clinic. Thanks to his treatment there, Brad says he now gets more sleep and better sleep than he ever has in his life. "I was super, super skeptical . . . but it worked really well," he tells me.

To be clear, it is true that some of us are more vulnerable to insomnia than others. Age, metabolism, and genetics are part of a long list of what are considered "predisposing factors" to insomnia. But Brad and I are perfect examples that being predisposed to insomnia does not mean insomnia is inevitable. So instead of throwing our hands up at the biological or psychological factors causing our insomnia, let's instead learn how to work with them to get our sleep back on track.

Insomnia vs. Sleep Deprivation

The terms *insomnia* and *sleep deprivation* are often used interchange-ably, but they're actually not the same thing. It's true that insomnia can cause sleep deprivation, but you can be sleep-deprived without having insomnia, and, perhaps more surprisingly—you can have insomnia without being sleep-deprived.

That's because insomnia is not about how much you sleep, it's about how efficiently you sleep. If you only get five hours of sleep every day, you are almost definitely sleep-deprived. But if that's because you only spend five hours in bed, you don't have insomnia. On the flip side, if you get eight hours of sleep every night, you're probably not sleep-deprived. But if you spend twelve hours in bed to get those eight hours of sleep, you are almost certainly an insomniac.

The importance of this distinction will become clear as you continue through the book.

Types of Insomnia

Difficulty falling asleep is called initial or onset insomnia, diffi-culty staying asleep is called middle or maintenance insomnia, and waking up too early is called late or terminal insomnia. You can have just one, two, or a combination of all three, like me. The next question is: How often do you experience this, and for how long?

"Chronic" vs. "Acute" Insomnia

The generally accepted threshold for when insomnia is considered chronic and in need of treatment is when it happens at least three days a week for at least three months.

Anything less than that is considered acute insomnia. The typical ad-vice for acute insomnia: Do nothing, it'll probably go away on its own.

But as evidenced by the aforementioned 10 to 60 percent of the population estimated to have chronic insomnia, sometimes it doesn't go away on its own. Also, I can't ignore a paper cut for five minutes. Are we really expected to ignore insomnia for three months and just hope it goes away? Is this really the best we can do?

Dr. Jason Ellis, director of the UK's Northumbria Centre for Sleep Research, says no. "There's no evidence to suggest that insomnia is insomnia [only] after three months," he tells me. "And there is a lot that we can do during that time."

Instead Ellis, who specializes in acute insomnia, says his cutoff is around two weeks. The occasional bad night or string of bad nights during a time of stress is perfectly normal. But Ellis says if your sleep problems have lasted beyond two weeks, they're no longer just a normal stress response—something is perpetuating them. And interventions can prove very helpful. For clarity's sake, I like to call this "established" insomnia.

A 2015 study that Ellis authored shows 60 percent of patients who received treatment for established insomnia were in remission within a month, compared to only 15 percent of those who didn't receive treatment. And a 2019 study he did involving prisoners showed 73 percent were in remission within a month of early intervention, even though none of their cases were considered chronic.

My mother has had insomnia for decades, and even she doesn't meet the technical definition for chronic insomnia, because she says it happens "at least once a week," not at least three days a week. But Mom checks every other box for chronic insomnia. "What bothers me is that sometimes I'm so, so tired. Oh my God, I just want to put my head down and go to sleep," she tells me. "And then, as I lay in bed, all of a sudden I wake up, and I can't fall asleep." This is something called conditioned arousal, a calling card of chronic insomnia, and a sign that your insomnia needs to be addressed. So whether it's been three months or three weeks, if your sleep issues have been going on long enough and consistently enough to really bother you—which they probably have if you're reading this book—it's time to take action.

Insomniac vs. Person with Insomnia

You'll notice throughout this book I sometimes use *insomniac* as shorthand for people with insomnia. It's a common term, but it's one many sleep experts hate, because they feel the term *insomniac* suggests that insomnia defines you. This is important because insomnia feeds on attention and performance anxiety. The more we worry about our sleep and tell ourselves that we're broken and can't sleep, the more likely we are to have trouble sleeping. So if calling yourself an insomniac cements those feelings for you, it can have a negative impact.

To me, however, the word *insomniac* conveys something different. When I was struggling, calling myself an *insomniac* was a subtle reminder that I was part of a huge group of people who are dealing with or have dealt with this very same problem, and that, like so many before me, I could get through this. I think this was an important realization for my recovery.

That said, I in no way consider insomnia a part of my identity and honestly never have. Even in the depths of my struggle, if I had been asked to give a short introduction of who I am, *insomniac* would not have been included in that description.

So please don't allow my use of this term throughout this book to make you think any differently about yourself or think that insomnia is now a part of who you are. Instead just realize that you have a temporary problem and an army of people, both doctors and patients, who understand exactly what you're going through and who can attest to the fact that it is fixable—if you use the right solutions.

Doctors and Sleeping Pills

Unfortunately, even doctors often don't know the right solutions for insomnia. According to Harvard Medical School, the most recent survey found four-year med schools on average provide "less than two hours of formal education directed at sleep" —including Harvard! This is why many primary care physicians (including mine, who's wonderful) often default to prescribing sleeping pills if a patient complains of trouble sleeping. They're trying to help, but they don't realize their prescription is at best a temporary solution and can actually make the problem worse. Even sleep experts who don't specialize in insomnia can make this mistake.

This is what happened to Whit Johnson, whose insomnia dates all the way back to middle school. "I would just lie in bed all night, and my brain would just eat away at me. I couldn't fall asleep. And as I got older, it got worse," he tells me. Whit says he got so sick of wasting time awake in bed that by his senior year in high school he just started getting up at four A.M. "I would go to Denny's all by myself. Then I would go from Denny's to the gym, I would work out, and then I would go to school," he says. By the time the school day ended, Whit says he was dragging, angry, and anxious.

As his issues continued through college and beyond, Whit saw sleep expert after sleep expert, who wrote him prescription after prescription. "I tried all sorts of medication. It was Ambien for a while. I tried Lunesta, some of the others. One psychiatrist even put me on an antipsychotic medication, like for people who have schizophrenia, to just really try to calm my brain at night. None of it worked," he says.

By the time he was anchoring morning news at KNBC in Los Angeles, Whit says he was "throwing down five cups of coffee" to stay awake, then taking Ambien to fall asleep, occasionally adding alcohol to the mix. But he realized something was really wrong when he started getting debilitating headaches. "It almost felt like a pop in the back of my neck, and then it would crawl forward through my skull, and I thought that I was having an aneurysm," he says.

The headaches led Whit to a sleep neurologist, who attributed them to a variety of factors including extreme lack of sleep and circadian rhythm issues from his overnight work schedule. But the neurologist said the primary culprit was likely Ambien. He gave Whit a few behavioral solutions that helped him get off Ambien and improved his sleep. Whit says he hasn't had those headaches since.

That's not to say that sleeping pills are the enemy. In some cases, they can play a helpful role in treating sleep disorders or other medical issues. But sleeping pills are rarely needed to treat insomnia. When they are used, they need to be managed thoughtfully, usually as a bridge to a long-term treatment, rather than as a lifelong solution. So if you're regularly taking sleeping pills—over-the-counter or prescription—you should be doing so under the guidance of a sleep specialist who specializes in your condition.

If you already regularly take sleeping pills and want to come off them, a sleep specialist can also offer guidance on how to do that safely.

The Truth About Sleep Hygiene

Your doctor might also suggest sleep hygiene to fix your insomnia. This is just a fancy way of saying good sleep habits and a good sleep environment. But trying to fix established insomnia with sleep hygiene is like trying to fix a cavity with dental hygiene—brush all you want, the cavity's not going anywhere. To fix insomnia that's already taken root, you'll need a different approach.

THE MYTH-BUSTING FIX:
FORGET SLEEP DEBT DOOM

It's easy to be terrified by the steady flow of scary headlines telling us insomnia is going to make us look terrible, feel terrible, and probably kill us. The truth is many of these warnings incorrectly use the term *insomnia* when they mean *sleep deprivation*—which, as explained above, are not the same thing. Equating insomnia and sleep deprivation is like equating a lack of appetite to starvation. Sure, we usually don't eat if we have no appetite, but that doesn't mean we're starving. Maybe we don't like the food available or our stomach is upset—or maybe we're already full!

Similarly, for reasons that will become clear in part 2, most insomniacs actually aren't that sleep deprived. Believe it or not, some aren't sleep deprived at all!

Many articles and books also incorrectly assume that because studies show people with insomnia are more likely to have other medical conditions, that means insomnia must be *causing* these illnesses. This is kind of like saying that because people who own ashtrays are more likely to have lung cancer, ashtrays must be causing lung cancer. Correlation is not causation. Considering all the obvious ways being sick can disrupt your sleep, it's entirely plausible that in many cases the sickness is actually causing the insomnia, not the other way around.

Regardless, even if you are experiencing symptoms from sleep deprivation, our bodies have an amazing ability to recover once we get our sleep back on track.

The most extreme example of this that I know of comes from HumanCo CEO Jason Karp. At twenty-three, Jason, an extreme overachiever, decided to boost his productivity by, among other things, teaching himself to speed-read and training himself to sleep less . . . a lot less. "I started reading some stuff from the military about how to go on very little sleep . . . and how to optimize using micronaps and caffeine," he tells me. "I was literally setting alarm clocks [for] two A.M., so that in case I fell asleep, I'd have to wake back up again."

The training worked. Jason, who usually needs at least seven hours of sleep, reduced his sleep to between two and four hours a night, then continued that for eight weeks. But his success came with consequences. "I was losing my hair in clumps. I had psoriasis plaques all over my body. The most problematic thing I had was I was losing my vision," he tells me.

Jason was diagnosed with a degenerative corneal disease and told he'd be blind by the age of thirty. As his problems mounted, he stayed up later and later, trying to learn as much as possible about each condition and figure out how to fix them. "Remember the beginning of *The Matrix* when they just show Neo scouring the internet looking for Morpheus, and he's in a dark room, and he's on his computer, and he's falling asleep? . . . I felt like that!" he says.

Jason also went to six or seven doctors to try to uncover what was happening to him, but none of them could figure it out. Not a single one asked him about his sleep or his diet. Then finally an endocrinologist ran a battery of tests on him and gave Jason his first clue. "You have the highest level of cortisol I've ever seen in a human being," the doctor told him. At that rate, the doctor said, Jason wouldn't live to see forty, maybe not even thirty-five. He added, "You should probably figure out what's causing all this stuff, because you have so many different diseases right now that there's no way they're not linked."

Through his research Jason was eventually able to connect cortisol to his skin condition, and his skin condition to his eye condition. And then he remembered another time that he had that skin condition. "I was pledging my fraternity, we had a hell weekend where they literally forced us to stay awake and just drink beer, and we couldn't eat food," he tells me. So Jason identified three possible culprits—lack of sleep, alcohol, and gluten (from the beer)—and resolved to stop drinking, eat a clean diet, and get more sleep. It took him a while to be able to sleep normally again, but within roughly six months, all his symptoms started to disappear.

Jason says, "I went to my doctor, who was a total prick, one of these really arrogant Park Avenue know-it-alls, who believed my disease was incurable. And I said, 'Hey, Doc, I actually cured my vision, I can see again!'"

The doctor assured Jason that wasn't possible, and to prove his point he measured Jason's corneas. The measurements had previously shown that Jason's eyes were increasingly cone-shaped, one of the main indications of his eye condition. But this time Jason's eyes were spherical again. His "incurable" condition had completely reversed itself! The doctor told Jason he'd never seen anything like it in his whole career.

It's important to note that Jason's problems didn't arise from insomnia. He *forced* himself to stay awake—two very different things. But even after years of being habitually sleep-deprived by about an hour and a half each day, and then all those weeks of extreme sleep deprivation, Jason still healed once he started sleeping well again.

Does this mean sleep debt isn't a serious issue? Of course not. Sleep is crucial to every aspect of our health, and the sooner you start getting enough of it, the better. But myth-busting this pervasive "sleep debt doom" narrative is an especially important first step for insomniacs, because the fear of the consequences of insomnia often perpetuate insomnia. So to start things off, let's all take a breath. We're going to be fine.

THE GROUNDWORK FIX:
VISIT YOUR DOCTOR

While, as mentioned above, your primary care physician is likely not well qualified to treat insomnia, it's still a good idea to visit your doctor. For starters, you'll want to ensure any interventions you're planning to try are safe for you. You'll also want to rule out any other conditions that might be causing or contributing to your sleep issues.

But contrary to popular belief, chronic insomnia that's caused by another condition often persists even after the primary condition is resolved. So unless your insomnia is very recent, consider addressing it *in addition to* addressing any underlying conditions. Not only will you enjoy relief from your insomnia, but you may find your sleep improvements help you recover from the underlying condition.

THE GOLD STANDARD FIX:
CBT-I

While it may not sound familiar, the actual gold standard treatment for chronic insomnia is cognitive behavioral therapy for insomnia, or CBT-I, administered by a behavioral sleep specialist. Unlike sleeping pills, which just treat the symptoms of insomnia, CBT-I targets the two main causes of insomnia—high arousal and low sleep drive—to actually cure it.

The downside is CBT-I requires more time and effort than just popping a pill, and the bigger problem is it requires regular visits with a behavioral sleep specialist, who can be hard to find and can have very long wait lists.

Part 2 of this book is largely based on the principles of CBT-I.

Digital CBT-I

While traditional CBT-I is like working out with a personal trainer, digital CBT-I is more like using a workout video at home. You won't get the accountability and truly tailored approach that comes from a dedicated sleep specialist, but research suggests it can still be effective for those who stick with it. Below are some of the pros and cons of some of the the more robust, peer-reviewed digital CBT-I options.

Somryst

Somryst was granted FDA authorization in 2020 as the first prescription digital therapeutic indicated to treat chronic insomnia in patients twenty-two or older. According to its parent company, the app uses algorithms to provide patients with tailored CBT-I over six to nine weeks. To use it you'll need a prescription from your doctor or you can go to Somryst.com to get an online prescription via a $45 telemedicine appointment. The irony is, because it requires a prescription, the app is off-limits to behavioral sleep psychologists, despite the fact that behavioral sleep psychologists developed most, if not all, of the methods the app is based on. Somryst also costs $900. For some this may be covered by insurance, others may qualify for discounts, but some may be stuck paying that out of pocket. The other potential downside is Somryst works via sleep restriction therapy, which is recommended for many but not all insomnia patients. More on sleep restriction and other alternatives in chapter 5.

Sleepio

Sleepio describes itself as a "tailored self-help system" that aims to teach users CBT-I techniques over a number of weekly sessions. The content is tailored to each user with the help of an algorithm, user input, and data from wearable devices. Unfortunately the program is only available in the United States through employers who choose to provide it as a benefit, or if you participate in a Sleepio study. You can check Sleepio.com for eligibility and lots of other helpful information.

CBT-i Coach

CBT-i Coach is described as "a mobile app for people who are engaged in CBT-I with a health provider, or who have experienced symptoms of insomnia and would like to improve their sleep habits." Developed by the U.S. Department of Veterans Affairs, Stanford University School of Medicine, and the U.S. Department of Defense, the app is available to veterans and civilians alike free of charge. CBT-i Coach has a lot of great features, but my personal favorite is the "Sleep Prescription" tool, which helps users with sleep restriction therapy by recommending specific bedtimes and wake-up times based on your entries in the app's Sleep Diary (more on sleep restriction in chapter 5). Even if you don't plan to do sleep restriction, this app can be a great tool to learn lots of CBT-I techniques proven to help people sleep better. But unfortunately CBT-i Coach is not as robust as the other options listed here.

BedTyme

BedTyme is a CBT-I-based app that aims to educate users about insomnia while offering daily guidance on how to fix it. It starts by asking you a number of questions, then forms a plan based on your answers. From there, the app gives you a short daily survey about your sleep and offers guidance on next steps. BedTyme was created by a sleep physician, Dr. Daniel Erichsen, and has stellar reviews in the App Store and on Google Play. It also includes access to your own personal sleep coach whom you can message for additional guidance, questions, or troubleshooting. But BedTyme has not been clinically tested, an important distinction from the options above, and at its current price tag of $129.99 a month, BedTyme isn't cheap. According to the app, most clients "graduate" in four to six weeks.

THE DIY FIX:
SELF-HELP

For those who don't have access to an adequate digital CBT-I option or a qualified behavioral sleep specialist, the Mayo Clinic points out that self-help alternatives like "CDs, books or websites on CBT techniques" may be beneficial. I'm living proof of that.

After my initial appointment with Dr. Jordan Stern from BlueSleep.com, he sent me home with two devices: one to test for sleep apnea, the other to analyze my sleep architecture. But the next morning I was asked to do standby anchor duty for *Good Morning America*. The schedule change threw me off and plunged me back into my one-to-three-hour sleep range. The sleep apnea test still worked and came back negative. But I was getting so little sleep that the sleep architecture test was basically useless. So Dr. Stern said to wait until I was back to my "normal" five hours of sleep to try the second test again.

To speed up that process, I sought out articles and books written by sleep clinicians and tried their various recommendations, based on my symptoms and circumstances, occasionally asking Dr. Stern for guidance along the way. My goal was to get back to five hours of sleep ASAP, so I could do the sleep architecture test again and start CBT-I. But to my surprise, my DIY approach worked so well, it didn't just get me back to five hours—it got me to a full "night's" sleep.

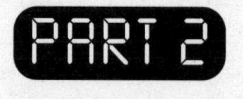

PART 2

SLEEP DRIVE VS.
AROUSAL

Imagine the best sleeper you know, the kind of person who's out within minutes of putting their head on the pillow. Someone who can sleep on planes and in cars. Someone who, despite feeling well rested, can enjoy an afternoon nap just because.

Now imagine someone put a gun to that person's head and ordered them to fall asleep within twenty minutes or else. They'd probably have a hard time. That's because anxiety or worry triggers an alerting response known as arousal, and arousal is a very powerful sleep killer. This, in a nutshell, is what insomnia is: a battle between arousal and your sleep drive—and arousal is winning.

I like to think of this as our Sleep Seesaw. Under ideal conditions, during the day our sleep drive is low and our wake drive is high, keeping our sleep seesaw in the awake position.

Awake

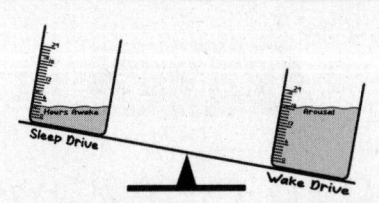

Then by bedtime our sleep drive is high and our wake drive is low, firmly planting our seesaw into the sleep position.

Asleep

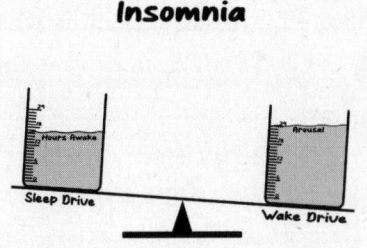

But the more aroused we are at bedtime, the more wake drive we build up. With enough arousal, our sleep drive can't compete, and our seesaw tips back into awake territory.

Insomnia

And you don't need a gun to your head to trigger arousal. For those of us predisposed to insomnia, even normal sources of stress, excitement, or mental activity can sometimes be enough. That arousal can also aggravate other sleep disorders, like RLS.

The most frustrating part is sleep effort itself is an arousal trigger. That's one of the reasons our hostage in the scenario above can't sleep: for once, they're trying really hard to. And in a cruel twist, the harder we try to sleep, the more we work ourselves up and the less likely sleep becomes. It's like we're putting the gun to our own head, which is useless because sleep isn't something we do—it's something that happens to us.

Still, that doesn't mean we're powerless against insomnia. As psychiatrist Dr. Nga Tran suggests, think of sleep as a guest we're inviting to a party. We can't force it to come, and the more desperate we are, the less likely it is to show up. But just as there are things we can do to make a party more enticing, we can create conditions that make it likely sleep will not only come but stay a while.

CHAPTER 3

Overactive Mind

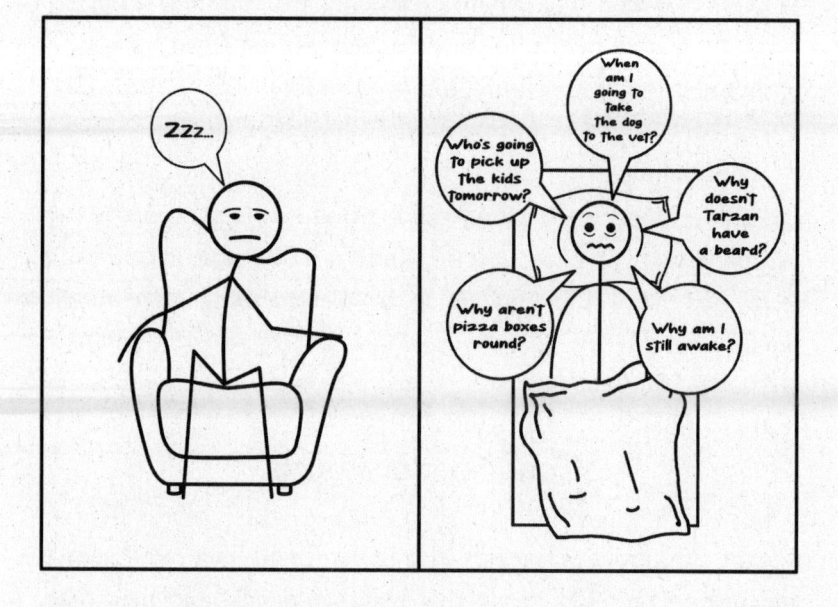

TRYING TO SLEEP WHEN WE have insomnia is like trying to sleep while someone is constantly pestering you with questions like "Are you asleep yet?" The obvious answer is "No, because you won't SHUT UP!" And the obvious solution is to get that person to go away. The problem is we are both the person trying to sleep *and* the annoying person asking all the questions. So the first thing we need to do is turn the volume down on that voice by dialing back our arousal.

In other words, we need to learn to relax. But if you've ever had someone tell you to "just relax" or "calm down," you know that's easier said than done.

The extra-tricky part is when we have insomnia, it can feel like arousal shows up out of nowhere—and at the worst times. My routine, for example, would often play out like this:

1. Start dozing off on the couch.
2. Head to bed (just a few feet away).
3. Suddenly feel wide awake.
4. Lie in bed worrying about not sleeping and thinking about everything from my to-do list, to a conversation I had, to what I should be for Halloween . . . in five months.

Sound familiar?

I always thought the act of walking from the living room to my bedroom was giving me a second wind. In reality, it wasn't the walk to the bed that was revving me up. It was something called conditioned arousal.

Conditioned Arousal

Conditioned arousal develops because our brain likes to anticipate and prepare. Eat something that makes you sick, and next time you're near it, you might feel nauseated at just the smell of that food. This happens because your brain makes the connection between that food and your sickness, and triggers that response to prevent you from eating it again. On the flip side, walk into your favorite restaurant and your mouth may start to water before you've even looked at the menu. Your brain has made a connection between that restaurant and food and is getting you ready to eat as soon as you walk in the door. This is called classical conditioning, or as I like to call it, mental autopilot.

Unfortunately, our mental autopilot can also kick in if we repeatedly get into bed, then do something mentally stimulating, like check emails, peruse social media, have emotional conversations, or think about something stressful. After a while, our brain starts to associate our bed with this mental arousal, and the act of getting into bed becomes a cue to automatically enter that mentally active state. Once we put down the phone or the crisis passes, and there's nothing else for our active mind to work on, it'll create its own work: by rehashing the past or worrying about the future.

From that point, it becomes a growing and vicious cycle. Thinking and worrying make it hard to fall asleep, which makes us worry about the fact that we're not sleeping. Then THOSE worries keep us awake. Eventually you might not even have to be in bed—just knowing it's bedtime can start to trigger those worries.

Imagine being exhausted all day yet being filled with dread the moment you realize you can finally go to bed! This was me. Of course it wasn't sleep I was dreading, but the act of lying in bed awake, frustrated, and endlessly cycling through negative thoughts.

So I handled this in the most mature and sensible way possible: avoidance. As soon as bedtime hit, I'd convince myself that I *had* to watch that TV show or organize my kitchen cabinets or shop for something online or research an idea—anything to avoid going to bed. It's worth noting that I didn't realize this was an avoidance tactic at the time. I genuinely felt I had to do these things urgently. Also, at least some of these activities could make for a good way to unwind before bed, but I wasn't doing them in a relaxing way. I was clinging somewhat obsessively to them, trying to keep my mind as active and occupied as possible so I wouldn't have to think about my bedtime anxiety. When I would finally give in and go to bed, I was exhausted, but my mind was racing. The later it was, the more anxiety I would have about how I wasn't going to get enough sleep.

Memory

Another reason for our barrage of often-repetitive bedtime thoughts has to do with memory. If I dictated an important phone number to you and you couldn't write it down, how would you remember it? You would probably repeat it to yourself over and over again. This is how our brain remembers things when it's given no better alternative. By repeatedly running over our to-do list and other thoughts, our mind is simply trying to ensure we don't forget these things. Unfortunately those reminders often keep us from sleeping, and what's one of the side effects of poor sleep? *Forgetfulness.* Thanks, mind!

No Mental Break

There's all sorts of complicated research that explains the benefits of mental downtime, but you don't need to be a scientist to understand why lack of downtime was hurting my sleep: my mind was cycling through thoughts in bed because I gave it no other option.

At the height of my insomnia, I was working ten P.M. to roughly nine A.M. for *World News Now, America This Morning,* and *Good Morning America.* I was so busy during those hours, on most days I wouldn't even stop to use the bathroom. In addition to that, I would often do shoots during the day for one of the above shows or *Nightline.* If I wasn't in bed or working, I'd be doing research, cooking, fixing something around the house, and/or devising my latest life hack (I'm obsessed). Even when I found time to get my nails done, I would listen to podcasts at the same time in hopes of getting a story idea. There wasn't a minute in which I wasn't actively thinking about or consuming information. No wonder my mind would start rehashing and analyzing when I finally tried to sleep—it was the only opportunity available.

Jason Karp had a similar experience. After his eight-week stint of forced sleep deprivation, it took him about six months to be able to sleep well again. He says part of the problem was his obsession with being productive. He would take notes while reading the newspaper, he barely made time for friends, and the only movies he'd watch were documentaries he wanted to learn from. "Everything was about self-advancement and self-improvement," he says.

In other words, Jason was driving himself to be mentally aroused all the time. And remember how he had super-high cortisol levels? Guess what fuels arousal? Cortisol, which is kind of like the slow-release form of adrenaline.

Jason eventually started seeing a therapist who described him as an "engine that's redlining constantly." And just like you can't throw a redlining engine into park, you can't expect a mind that's so aroused to suddenly fall asleep. First, you have to learn to slow down.

The Threat of Wakefulness

Unfortunately for insomniacs, our conditioned arousal often goes beyond just cycling through to-do list items or processing our day. Instead, our fear of being awake kicks our arousal into overdrive. We spin scary narratives as we lie in bed about how terrible our day will be without sleep, how we won't be able to function, how we might get sick. Sometimes I even worried I would die from sleep deprivation.

This might sound extreme, but we're actually more prone to catastrophic thinking after bedtime.

As Dr. Jason Ellis explains in his book, *The One-Week Insomnia Cure,* some parts of the brain that downregulate while we sleep will still downregulate at their usual times even if we're awake—including "the part of the brain that covers rationality, reasoning and logic." So we may be awake overnight, but our reason and logic are basically still asleep. Notice a new freckle during the day, and you might make a note to see the dermatologist. Start thinking about that freckle overnight and you could find yourself planning your own funeral . . . even though there's no evidence it's anything more than a freckle.

Now consider that insomniacs have a general tendency to be awake after bedtime and to obsess over the consequences of not sleeping, and you can start to see how this plays out. As we repeatedly lie in bed catastrophizing about how doomed we are, we send our brains a clear message: being awake after bedtime is a serious threat. After a while, as bedtime approaches, our brain prepares us to face this threat, the same way it helps us face any threat—by triggering hyperarousal, aka our fight-or-flight response. Our heart rate and breath might speed up, our muscles get more tense, our pupils dilate to take in more light. This is all helpful when we need to be alert in the face of danger, but it's very unhelpful if we're trying to sleep.

To make matters worse, typical sleep advice often reinforces this. I can't tell you how many times I've heard that if I have trouble sleeping, I should read a boring book. Some even advise reading an instruction manual. Since boredom generally facilitates sleep, the logic is that you can basically bore yourself to sleep. But this approach ignores an alternative reaction to boredom: frustration.

ABC News correspondent Trevor Ault says he tried this strategy by listening to deliberately boring podcasts aimed at lulling the listener to sleep. "That was a horrific failure," Trevor says. "I just kept thinking about why it was a terrible story. Because we're professional storytellers, so I'm like, oh, man, you got to cut this out and trim the fat here." Instead of feeling sleepy, Trevor said he ended up feeling frustrated over the crappy story and even more awake, thinking of all the ways he could fix it.

My friend Brad had a similar experience when he tried his doctor's suggestion to fold laundry when he couldn't sleep. Since Brad hates folding laundry, it just made him feel pissed off. "For me folding laundry isn't calming . . . it would fully wake me up. Because I'd be like, okay, this is something that I have to do."

Dr. Jason Ong, a clinician and researcher with Northwestern University's Center for Circadian & Sleep Medicine, recalls a patient who said he read a phone book anytime he woke up overnight. Unlike Trevor and Brad, this patient felt the boring task did help him to fall back asleep, but when Ong asked if he found the activity soothing and relaxing, the guy replied, "No, I hate myself for having to read the phone book to fall asleep."

So even if it works in the moment, if the boredom strategy leaves you frustrated, it can still backfire. Because now you have yet another source of sleep anxiety: "I have to sleep, otherwise I'll have to read the effing phone book!"

The more reasons we give ourselves to fear wakefulness, the more we see it as a threat, and the more likely we are to go into a state of hyperarousal as we prepare for sleep.

The Sleep Through the Night Myth

While we've been led to believe that a good night's sleep means sleeping straight through from bedtime to wake-up time, that's actually not how human sleep works. Instead, we sleep in cycles, going through sleep stages that get increasingly deeper, followed by REM sleep, in which we do most of our dreaming. After 70 to

100 minutes (not exactly 90, as many articles and books claim), one cycle ends and a new one begins. But here's the interesting part: in between the cycles we usually wake up. And I don't just mean we insomniacs, I mean *everybody*.

Most people just fall right back asleep so quickly they don't even remember these awakenings—hence the feeling that they "slept through the night." Insomniacs, on the other hand . . . we basically freak out.

As sleep physician Dr. Daniel Erichsen explains, "When somebody with insomnia wakes up for whatever reason, they become aware of being awake, they react to being awake, they go, 'Dang it, I'm awake!' Then the thoughts go into 'Why am I awake? What happened? How can I change this? I need to sleep!' And then you become fully awakened."

It's not the fact that we wake up throughout the night that's the problem. It's the fact that our worries create arousal, which in turn keeps us awake. So the next time you hear the term *sleep through the night*, including in this book, please know it's a loose expression. And the next time it's two A.M. and you're wondering why you're awake, it might be helpful to remember the answer is probably because that's completely normal.

The Myth of the "Quiet Mind"

When I was dealing with conditioned arousal, I had no idea what it was, so I described it like so many insomniacs do: "I can't sleep because I can't shut off my brain." This is an accurate description of what conditioned arousal feels like. But it highlights a major misconception we insomniacs seem to share: that the rest of the world somehow turns off their thoughts in order to fall asleep.

For me, it didn't help that mindful meditation had just become the new it trend. I was constantly seeing articles and TV segments touting how meditation "quiets the mind." That's exactly what I needed! So I downloaded a meditation app and, as always, kept my expectations super realistic: after one session I would be like Neo from *The Matrix*, stopping my thoughts like slow-motion bullets.

The reality went more like this:

Meditation app narrator: *Focus on the breath. Feel your stomach expand and relax . . .*

Me: *Got it. The breath, focusing on the breath. Breathe in, breathe out. Man, I am nailing this!*

App dude: *Now bring your attention down to your feet. Observe any sensations in your toes . . .*

Me: *Focusing on my feet. Do I feel any sensations in my toes? I don't think so. But that reminds me, I forgot to get those gel insoles I wanted for my sneakers again. Damn it, I suck! Maybe they sell them at the pharmacy and I can just grab them on my way to work.*

App dude: *Slowly move your attention to your ankles . . .*

Me: *Idiot! Stop thinking about insoles! Ankles . . . focus on the ankles. Breathe in, breathe out. Ankles feel fine. Breathe in, breathe out. My shins are tight, though. Breathe in, breathe out. They always feel a bit achy. Wonder if the insoles would help with that? Maybe I should just order them online so I don't forget. I wonder if they have them on Amazon Prime?*

App dude: *Observe any sensations throughout the leg . . .*

Me: *Amazon Prime? Seriously, Diane?! You're supposed to be meditating and you're thinking about Amazon PRIME?!!! Get it together!*

I'm not sure I even made it to the torso before I finally gave up. I was hoping to find this peaceful place of quiet, sleep-filled Zen. Instead, I was even more awake than usual and super mad at myself. Not only was I a crappy sleeper, with crappy uncushioned sneakers—now I was also a crappy meditator.

But the real reason I failed was because I was trying to achieve the impossible. As my colleague Dan Harris, author of *10% Happier* and *Meditation for Fidgety Skeptics*, explains, "This is the most pernicious misconception around meditation . . . drop the idea of clearing your mind. That is impossible unless you're enlightened or you have died." (More on meditation in chapter 20.)

And just as meditators don't clear their minds, neither do good sleepers. As clinical psychologist Dr. Nick Wignall explains, "Your brain is always incredibly active, even when you're sleeping." Wignall says when we do fall sleep, it's not because our thoughts go quiet. It's because "your sleep drive outcompetes your level of arousal."

But when we buy into the myth of the quiet mind, we create our own problem. Our worries about thinking and our efforts to stop thinking just increase our mental arousal and make it harder for our sleep drive to compete.

THE "ARE YOU SERIOUS?" FIX:
CONSTRUCTIVE WORRY

My first sleep breakthrough came when I realized I didn't need to distract myself or silence my thoughts and feelings. Instead I needed to embrace and process them in a productive (and idiotproof) way. Enter constructive worry. It's just a simple practice of writing all your worries on one side of a page and the next steps to solving them on the other, and I have to admit, when I first read about it, I couldn't help but roll my eyes. Ambien didn't put me to sleep anymore, but a dressed-up to-do list was going to help?

Now when people ask how I beat insomnia, constructive worry is the first thing I mention. I love this technique for so many reasons: It's cheap (just need a notebook and a writing utensil), it takes only a few minutes, it's super straightforward, so you don't have to worry about "doing it wrong," and most importantly, it works! Here's why:

- By thinking through your worries *before* bed, you decrease the need to think about them *in* bed.
- By doing this regularly, you create a new association: your brain starts to realize *this* is the time for worry, not when you're in bed.
- The nature of the exercise helps to shift your focus to solutions, rather than ruminating on problems. This can help with sleep and also ease general feelings of anxiety or depression and make you feel less stuck.
- By writing your worries down, you remove the need for your brain to remind you to deal with them. You can relax knowing you won't forget—because they're right there on the page.

Jason Karp does an abbreviated version of this which he calls his brain dump. "I write every single thing down that's in my head. Whether it's 'Remember to call this guy in the morning, remember to do this, remember to do that,' or it could be just an idea that's percolating," he says. Since Jason's biggest problem was waking up in the middle of the night, firing on all cylinders, he wanted to ensure any thought that might occur to him at two A.M. was already on the page. He says, "When I started doing that religiously, I started sleeping so much better."

But, as with any other tool in this book, it's important to enjoy constructive worry for its own benefits. Doing anything with the intention of making sleep happen usually results in us putting more pressure on ourselves to sleep, which backfires. So avoid getting in the mindset of "Okay, I did constructive worry. Now let's see if I sleep." Instead, try to think to yourself, "I did constructive worry. Now I feel less anxious."

How-To: Constructive Worry

Pick a time when you can do this every day—ideally a few hours before bed.

1. Get a notebook and draw a line to divide the page into two columns or use two pages side by side.
2. On the left side, list anything that's worrying you. On the right side, next to each worry, write the very next step to resolving that problem.

    -   If you don't know the fix, the next step might be to call someone for advice or research how to resolve it.
    -   If the problem has no resolution—because it can't be resolved, is out of your control, or because you're worried about something hypothetical—the next step might be to accept and move on. Write that too.

3. When you go to bed, keep the notebook nearby. If your worries return, remind yourself that you've figured out how to deal with them, and there's nothing else you can do for the day.

Adjustments

As with any technique in this book, you do not have to do constructive worry perfectly for it to work. *The best sleep solutions are the ones you'll actually do,* so make them work for you!

For example, I did not do this a few hours before bed as is recommended. My work schedule varies dramatically from day to day, so remembering to consistently block off time for constructive worry hours before bed is not happening. Instead, I store the notebook in my nightstand and do my constructive worry sitting on the bed, just before I brush my teeth and otherwise get ready to go to sleep. This technically betrays the cardinal rule: bed is for sleep and sex, nothing else. But I make sure I'm sitting on top of the covers, my back's against the headboard, etc. This is different enough from when I'm lying in bed, under the covers, head on the pillow, lights out, that my mind is able to differentiate between constructive worry time and sleep time. Jason says he did the same, and it still worked for him too.

After two weeks I no longer needed the daily constructive worry routine. My brain got the message: head on pillow does not mean it's time to think—it means it's time to sleep. But that notebook is still in my nightstand, and if I have a lot on my mind before bed or if I wake up stressed in the middle of the night, I still use it. If the hubs is already sleeping, I just slip out to the living room and write my list there. Usually just a few short minutes of jotting things down and I'm able to relax, let those thoughts go, and drift off to sleep.

Pro Tip: Love Your Notebook

Any notebook and pen will do, but I suggest using ones that, in the words of Marie Kondo, spark joy for you. Do you like the way the notebook looks? Do you like the way it feels in your hands? Do you like the spacing of the lines, or do you prefer no lines? Do you like the way the pen looks, feels, and writes? It's not crucial and doesn't have to be expensive (my notebook and pen are from the drugstore), but if seeing and holding that book and that pen give you pleasant feelings, it makes the whole process that much more enjoyable and easier to stick with.

THE WORD VOMIT FIX:
JOURNALING

Another way your notebook can help you sleep is journaling. I use this only when I'm dealing with something especially stressful.

How-To: Journaling

Put pen to paper and just write whatever you're thinking and feeling. Don't worry about the quality of the writing or if it even makes sense. Just let your stream of consciousness flow out of your head and blurt it out onto the page. If you're having trouble getting started, begin by completing the sentence "I can't sleep because . . . "

Journaling is generally much more productive than relentlessly trying to distract yourself from your worries, because, as I learned the hard way, once you turn the distraction off, your worries are still right there waiting for you. For me, journaling helps me sort out exactly what I feel about a given situation and why I feel that way. Since my mind always wants to figure things out and put them in order, this ability to make sense of my emotions allows my mind to stop dwelling on them.

To be clear, when I'm done journaling, I still feel those emotions. But because I understand where they're coming from, I can just accept them and let them hang out in the background instead of feeling consumed by them.

As a bonus, if you journal overnight, then read your words over the next day, you may notice your catastrophic worries that felt almost certain at night seem ludicrous in the light of day. If so, the next time you have those kinds of worries during the night, you can remind yourself that, like last time, you're probably just catastrophizing, and the situation is likely nowhere near as bad as it feels in this moment. It may not even be bad at all.

Gratitude Journal

Another journaling technique recommended for sleep is to take fifteen minutes before bed to write about how a recent positive experience made you feel, or to keep a gratitude journal where you just write down what you're thankful for. This can help you go to bed thinking about good things instead of all your worries.

THE LAZY FIX:
DO LESS

Ask a good sleeper what they do to drift off to sleep, and they usually just shrug. Because they don't do anything. But ask an insomniac, and you're likely to get a long list: screen-time curfews, caffeine curfews, herbal tea, essential oils, hot baths, stretches, breath work . . . all the things you typically see in sleep articles.

On the surface, this approach sounds sensible. These things are generally good for sleep. The problem is the *attitude* they create toward sleep is not, especially if you have insomnia. As Dr. Nick Wignall explains, "The implicit message . . . is that there's lots of stuff you need to do, think about, remember, and generally strive for if you want to be a successful sleeper."

It can also feel like we're giving ourselves an elaborate to-do list before bed, instead of winding down. Wignall says that as a result, our brain thinks to itself, *Well, I thought it was time to sleep, but . . . I'd better go back into work mode.*

So if your herbal tea, essential oil, and screen-time curfew make you happy and relaxed, great! If not, skip them. And go back to doing whatever you did before you had sleep problems. If keeping a sleep diary is making you more obsessive about sleep, ditch that too.

After your insomnia improves, if you want to try these things again to see if they make your sleep even better, go for it. But if you have conditioned arousal, right now the main thing keeping you from sleeping is worrying about not sleeping. And anything that adds to those worries is likely to do more harm than good.

THE TURNING THE TABLES FIX: ENJOY YOUR AWAKE TIME

One of the keys to falling asleep is to stop worrying about being awake, and one of the easiest ways to do that is to start enjoying your awake time. So if you can't sleep at night, get out of bed and try constructive worry, but plan some enjoyable activities you can do if you don't feel sleepy after that. You can read a good book, listen to a podcast, even (gasp!) watch TV—pretty much anything you find relaxing that doesn't involve bright light, cardio, big meals, caffeine, booze, drugs, and maybe video games. (More on these things later.) Do this until you feel sleepy, then go back to bed.

This might take a little experimenting to see what works for you. While most people find reading helps them wind down, my friend Brad found his usual books were too stimulating for him. "I would want to keep reading them . . . and then I just stay up until three-thirty in the morning reading a book," he tells me. After some trial and error, Brad, who loves to cook, found reading cookbooks was a nice sweet spot between engaging and relaxing. "It's not overly mentally stimulating, but [having] something I can actually read and focus on allowed me to kind of unwind and have my brain wind down. That absolutely helped me go back into bed at a lower velocity than I would have been mentally before," he tells me.

If you think of sleep as an invite to your party, this is like also inviting other people that you and sleep *both* like to hang out with. Not only does this make it a more tempting party for sleep to attend, but you'll also be more relaxed about whether or not sleep comes, and you'll enjoy yourself either way.

The less we fear being awake, the less pressure we put on ourselves to fall asleep, the less aroused we become, and the more likely sleep is to show up.

If you're someone like Jason Karp, who's always trying to be productive, this "enjoy your wake time" Fix also applies during your normal awake hours: find time in your day to do something for pure enjoyment. Jason says in his case that instruction came directly from his therapist, and his girlfriend at the time was more than happy to help. "We watched *Sex and the City*, and we watched silly romance movies, and we played video games where there wasn't any goal of getting good at something," he says.

For Jason, this was actually difficult, because the voice in his head would constantly criticize him for wasting time, but eventually he learned to appreciate the value of downtime. He explains, "When I started to embrace that there's a role of play just for the sake of play, and there's a role of enjoyment just for the sake of enjoyment . . . that started to quiet me down, because now before bed, I wasn't picking up a book that could make me better in any way. I was picking up a book I would just enjoy."

THE IGNORE IT FIX:
CARRY ON

Part of what feeds our sleep anxiety and arousal is attention. Insomnia LOVES attention. So do your best to deny it that reward.

I stumbled on this strategy by accident when I just randomly decided one day, *No matter what happens with my sleep, I'm going to just carry on as if everything's fine.* At the time I didn't know I was touching on something important. I was just fed up with spending all my time and energy thinking about and being miserable over my sleep. But it turns out when we stop focusing on our sleep and start focusing on other enjoyable things, we see that we can still live our lives, even after a bad night. This helps to take the pressure off, which in turn helps lower our arousal.

THE RECOGNIZABLE FIX:
RELAXATION TOOLS

There are a number of techniques aimed specifically at relaxation, from progressive muscle relaxation to breath work to various forms of meditation. I found these tools to be effective only after I incorporated the techniques above first. But again, what is relaxing will differ from person to person. If you want to try more traditional relaxation tools at this stage, go for it—just read chapter 20 before you do. As I learned the hard way, these tools can backfire on insomniacs due in part to our own misconceptions. The information in chapter 20 will help.

CHAPTER 4

Sleep Confidence and Misperception

SLEEP CONFIDENCE IS JUST THE confidence of knowing we're going to fall asleep when we go to bed, and it plays a big role in whether or not we do. People who fall asleep easily don't even think about sleep confidence—they just have it. But if you've been stuck in the cycle described in the previous chapter, chances are your sleep confidence is shot.

The problem is insomniacs are notoriously bad at judging our own sleep. We tend to overestimate how long it takes us to fall asleep and underestimate our total sleep—often by well over an hour! So we might be feeling terrible about our sleep when we're actually not sleeping that badly. In extreme cases this is classified as paradoxical insomnia, which is when we report having severe insomnia, but when measured objectively, our sleep looks fairly normal.

I know from my first sleep test, which happened right after a scheduling change, that my sleep at that time was objectively very poor. But I also now wonder how much of my problem was a product of misperception. One incident that sticks out is when I was convinced I went five days without any sleep right around my thirtieth birthday. It's what finally drove me to see my doctor and start taking Ambien. Now I realize I was likely suffering from a combination of insomnia AND sleep misperception. Had my primary care physician known more about sleep, she would have spotted my complaint of days without sleeping as a red flag for sleep misperception and immediately referred me to an insomnia specialist, instead of prescribing sleeping pills.

Note that insomniacs who have this issue aren't just making things up or imagining things. Instead, the leading theory on sleep misperception is that our heightened arousal, which continues during sleep, makes our brain much more active than a sleeping brain normally would be. It's like our sleep seesaw is still in sleep territory but hovering just slightly off the ground. This can make sleep feel a lot like being awake.

Misperceived Sleep

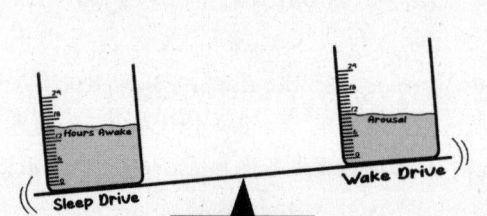

Because our brains are so active, we might also remember more of our time in bed than a normal sleeper would. This can make it feel like it took us longer to fall asleep and allow us to recall normal overnight awakenings we would otherwise forget.

My own additional hypothesis is that this kind of sleep does deplete our sleep drive, so we don't wake up *sleepy*, but because our brains were so active all night, we do wake up *tired*. More on that important distinction in the next chapter.

The good news is that just being aware of a misperception can help correct it and can also help our sleep confidence. So use the Fixes below to get a better objective picture of your sleep.

Hopefully you're pleasantly surprised with the amount of sleep you're actually getting, and if not, don't worry. Lowering arousal will help (see chapter 3). So will the tools in the next chapter—and your findings from this chapter will help you implement them.

THE HIGH-TECH FIX:
SLEEP ON CUE HACK

The Sleep On Cue app wasn't specifically designed for this purpose, but with a small work-around, it can be an easy, affordable way to gauge sleep onset and sleep misperception.

How-To: Sleep On Cue Hack

1. Purchase and download the Sleep On Cue App (currently $4.99).
2. Write down, on average, how long you think it takes you to fall asleep at bedtime. If you've been keeping a sleep diary, use the average of a week's worth of entries.
3. When you're ready to go to sleep, open Sleep On Cue and choose the "Take a Custom Nap" option.
4. Do a "practice" to ensure the tones are loud enough to hear when you're awake, but quiet enough not to wake you if you're sleeping, then hit "I'm ready for my nap."
5. Set both number pulldowns to 500 minutes and hit "OK."

   • If trying to gauge sleep onset after waking overnight, you may be able to choose the number of minutes until your wake time instead.

6. Find a comfortable sleeping position that allows you to have one hand on the phone and give the phone a nudge or shake every time you hear the tone until you fall asleep.
7. After the 500 minutes are done, the app will tell you how long it took you to fall asleep. Take a screenshot of this or log it for your records—the app will not save this info.

   • If you wake up before the 500 minutes are up, let the app continue to run in the background. It will give you your sleep onset time only after those 500 minutes are up.

(continued on next page)

8. Your average time after a week will give you an idea of your average sleep latency. Compare that to the number from step 1 to give you a general idea of your sleep misperception.
9. If you feel like you're awake longer than usual and getting frustrated, get out of bed and do something relaxing—but keep the app going for a few minutes and listen for more tones. If you don't hear any, it likely means you did fall asleep and then woke up again. Keep the app running to see when it predicts you fell asleep. You might also consider using the app's "Sleep Training" option for an hour or so the next night. The downside is it will wake you up if you do fall asleep; the upside is it will give you a much clearer sense of whether you're falling asleep without realizing it. (More on sleep training in the next chapter.)

THE CREATIVE FIX:
THE TISSUE TEST

The tissue test is my own adaptation of the spoon test, and another way to get an idea of how long it takes you to fall asleep. To do this you'll need a video camera with the ability to record in the dark (like a baby monitor or security camera) and a tissue.

How-To: The Tissue Test

1. Write down, on average, how long you think it takes you to fall asleep at bedtime. If you've been keeping a sleep diary, you can use the average of a week's worth of entries.
2. Set up a camera to capture video of you as you fall asleep. Make sure you'll see your hand and the floor in the shot. Hit record before you get in bed for the night.
3. Find a comfortable sleeping position that allows you to hold a tissue in your hand over the side of the bed, then go to sleep.
4. When you wake up, check the video to see how long it took for you to drop the tissue after you closed your eyes to fall asleep.
5. Use the average time over a week to give you an idea of your average sleep latency. Compare that to the number from step 1 to give you a general idea of your sleep misperception.

6. If it feels like you're awake longer than usual and you start to get frustrated, get out of bed, do something relaxing, and try again when you feel sleepier. If you get this feeling but notice the tissue is on the floor, it likely means you did fall asleep but just didn't realize it.

7. If you wake up in the middle of the night, you can do the test again when you come back to bed to gauge how long it takes you to fall back asleep.

8. If you go the whole night awake and never drop the tissue, contact a sleep specialist.

THE DUAL PURPOSE FIX:
AUDIOBOOK/PODCAST TEST

Listening to an audiobook or podcast at bedtime can have dual benefits when you're struggling with insomnia.

First, audiobooks or podcasts can serve as an effective distraction to stop us from thinking about sleep while we're lying in bed. This can help lower our arousal and help us fall asleep.

I still do this if I happen to break my own rule and read a problematic email near bedtime. To keep myself from endlessly troubleshooting the problem in my head, I put on an interesting podcast. I get sucked into the content, forget about the problem, and eventually fall asleep.

But in addition to that, a podcast or audiobook can also serve as an unofficial method of gauging how quickly we fall asleep. I've creatively named this the Audiobook/Podcast Test, which I put together with the help of Dr. Jade Wu.

How-To: Audiobook/Podcast Test

Before Going to Bed

1. Write down how long you think it usually takes you to fall asleep at bedtime. If you've been keeping a sleep diary, you can use the average of a week's worth of entries.
2. Leave a pen and notebook on your nightstand.
3. Choose any podcast or audiobook that you find interesting and engaging . . . just maybe not something with jump scares.
4. Set a sleep timer for the amount of time you think it usually takes to fall asleep plus an extra 30 minutes to give yourself a buffer.

Optional: If you share your bed or room, consider using a headphone headband or any other headphones you can comfortably sleep in.

Once in Bed

5. Play your podcast or audiobook, close your eyes, and enjoy.
6. If you're awake when the audio stops, make a tally mark in your notebook at that moment. The following night add an extra 30 minutes to your sleep timer.
7. If you wake up, the audio's stopped, and you don't see a tally mark—you likely fell asleep before your sleep timer ended.
8. The next day, quickly scan through the audio to find the last point you remember hearing the night before. This is likely when you fell asleep. Write down how far from your starting point this was.
9. After a week, compare your average results from step 8 to the number from step 1 to give you a general idea of your sleep misperception.
10. If you continuously are awake when the book or podcast ends, scan the audio. If you find any sections you don't remember, you were probably sleeping during that time. Count this when estimating your total sleep time.
11. If you estimate you're sleeping less than five hours a night, contact a sleep specialist.

Note: If you feel the audio is making it harder for you to sleep, ditch it, get out of bed, do something relaxing, and go back to bed when you feel sleepier. You can opt to try again with a different podcast/book, or ditch the technique altogether. It may not be right for you, and that's okay!

To be clear, there's no specific research on this method, but Dr. Wu, a sleep scientist and clinical psychologist at Duke University School of Medicine, tells me she's also found it to be effective—in both her personal and her clinical experience. "When people listen to an audiobook or podcast and they put on a sleep timer for say, thirty minutes, they often realize the next day that they must have fallen asleep faster than they thought because they didn't remember the last ten minutes of that book," she says, ". . . so it's sometimes really reassuring for people."

THE MIDDLE INSOMNIA FIX:
THE TALLY TEST

If you struggle with multiple overnight awakenings, try the Tally Test.

How-To: The Tally Test

1. Write down how many times you think you wake up overnight on average. If you've been keeping a sleep diary, you can use the average of a week's worth of entries.
2. Leave a pen and notebook on your nightstand.
3. Every time you wake up during the night quickly make a tally mark in the notebook.
4. After a week, compare your average number of tallies with your number from step 1 to gauge your level of misperception.

Optional: Combine this with any of the methods above to gauge how long it takes you to fall back asleep.

Note: Dr. Jason Ellis suggests using your mobile phone for this and dialing a star or hash every time you wake up. I find a notebook and a pen faster and easier. It also eliminates the temptation to do other things with my phone. Choose whichever option works best for you.

CHAPTER 5

Not Sleepy Enough

HAVE YOU EVER TRIED TO put a baby to sleep after a quick unplanned car nap? Spoiler alert: it sucks. The few minutes of crappy car sleep doesn't satisfy their sleep needs, but it does shave off just enough sleepiness to keep them from falling back asleep at home. The baby ends up tired but awake—and cranky. The same thing can happen to adults.

To understand why, you have to understand sleep drive, which luckily is as straightforward as understanding hunger. The longer we go without eating, the hungrier we become; then as we eat, our hunger dissipates. Same with sleep drive. The longer we're awake, the more the biochemical adenosine accumulates in our brain, which makes us sleepy. Then as we sleep, the adenosine dissipates, taking sleepiness with it. When we wake up, the process starts all over again.

Sleep Drive

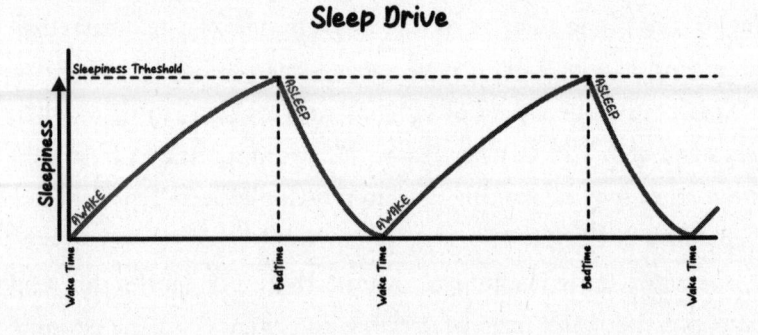

To borrow an analogy from baby sleep expert Cara Dumaplin, think of sleep drive like a "tired tank." Just as your car can't go the distance without enough gasoline in the gas tank, you can't fall asleep or stay asleep without enough adenosine in your "tired tank."

But while your car won't automatically drive itself and your body won't automatically feed itself, in a way sleep is more like breathing: you can hold your breath to a point, but eventually your body will automatically breathe for you. The same is true for sleep. There are many ways we can keep ourselves awake, but if your sleep drive gets high enough, eventually the body will take over and you will sleep—whether you like it or not.

One famous example of this is when Arianna Huffington suddenly collapsed at her desk and broke her cheekbone. In her book *The Sleep Revolution,* she describes how, to accommodate her demanding schedule, she had been allowing herself only three to four hours of sleep a night. "My body just couldn't take it anymore, and down I went, coming back to consciousness in a pool of blood," she writes.

Jason Karp says when he was sleeping two to four hours a night, the same would happen to him. "There were times that I would just fall asleep," he tells me. He still remembers one episode vividly. He took a rare break from productivity to go to a big Knicks game with his best friend. "It was a six P.M. tip-off, it wasn't even night, and I was out cold within five minutes of the game starting," he says. Jason's friend couldn't believe it. "He woke me up and he's like, 'Are you insane? Are you literally falling asleep at six P.M. in the middle of a loud basketball game?!' And I said, 'I didn't even realize I was asleep!'"

This is just one aspect of why it's so dangerous to drive when sleep-deprived, and another reason it's so important to treat conditions that may be making you unknowingly sleep-deprived, like sleep apnea or RLS.

But while most insomniacs assume that, like Huffington and Karp, our tired tank must be overflowing, chances are the opposite is true. Despite how tired we feel, our sleep drive is likely depleted. And the main reason is because we're following typical sleep advice.

The Eight-Hour Sleep Myth

How many times have you read or heard about the "recommended eight hours of sleep"? Type that phrase into Google and you'll see the number of articles containing it are endless. But the idea that we all need the same amount of sleep to be well rested is like saying we all need the same amount of food to be full: it's just not true.

The most general recommendation from the National Sleep Foundation is that most adults under sixty-four get somewhere between seven and nine hours of sleep a night. That's a pretty broad range. Keep reading, and you'll see those recommendations get even broader, with the foundation suggesting that as few as six hours or as many as ten "may be appropriate"—up to eleven if you're under twenty-five. If you're over sixty-four, anywhere from five to nine hours "may be appropriate." Scientists have even discovered gene mutations that cause a rare group of people to need only four to six hours.

Simply put, sleep needs vary greatly from person to person. Summing all of that up by suggesting eight hours is the recommended amount of sleep for everyone can be destructive.

For people who need more than eight hours, like my husband, targeting eight hours can leave them sleep-deprived. They and others might also mistake their sleepiness for laziness because they got the supposed recommended amount of sleep.

For people who need less than eight hours, like me, the eight-hour myth can also have consequences, because our sleep drive will let us get only so much sleep, just like our stomach size will let us eat only so much food. And the more time we spend in bed trying to force sleep, the more likely we are to develop conditioned arousal (chapter 3).

Orthosomnia

Our cultural obsession with eight hours has even contributed to a new sleep condition dubbed orthosomnia. This is when people become so obsessed with getting the perfect amount of sleep that their stress over not meeting that goal essentially gives them insomnia. This is often exacerbated by the use of sleep trackers.

Dan Harris, former co-anchor of the weekend edition of *Good Morning America,* experienced this firsthand, ironically after interviewing a sleep expert for his podcast *Ten Percent Happier.* Among other things, Dan says, the expert warned that if you don't get at least seven hours of sleep every night, you are in danger. Dan became fixated. "I got really focused on the idea that seven is the absolute minimum . . . and I was wearing the Oura Ring and seeing that I wasn't getting that," he tells me. From there, he says, things turned into "a mess."

Luckily, a few months later Dan interviewed a different sleep expert, Dr. Donn Posner. On the podcast, Posner told Dan that it's not about getting at least seven hours, it's about getting as much sleep as you need to "feel fine" the next day. He also very thoughtfully added that it's completely normal to feel sleepy right after we wake up, in the middle of the day when our circadian rhythm takes a dip, and at night when our sleep drive is high from having been awake all day. So the question is, do you feel fine the rest of the day?

Dan tells me, "Talking to Donn Posner had a really helpful effect on me, which was that I realized the true measure is 'How are you feeling?' And that just relaxed me a lot."

Dan says he still keeps a rough gauge of how much sleep he gets, but he primarily focuses on whether he feels like he needs a nap all day or has good energy, not on how many hours he got. "That has brought the temperature down in a way that's helped my sleep," he says.

In my case, the eight-hour myth had me reevaluating my entire history with sleep. As I complained about my insomnia to my husband and my doctor, I would often say things like, "I've had insomnia my whole life," or "I've always had trouble sleeping."

Now as I look back, I see that there were many occasions in my teens and early twenties where I was sleep-deprived because I decided studying, working, partying, or pretty much anything else was more important than sleeping. But I can't remember many where I tried to sleep at night but couldn't. Most of the time I slept fine and felt fine. As Mom knew all those years ago, I just didn't need eight hours.

Sleeping In and Napping

Whether you're aiming for eight hours or not, when you don't get the amount of sleep you were hoping for, it's easy to feel like you have to make up for that somehow—especially given how often we hear about the detrimental effects of sleep debt. So insomniacs often aim to recover sleep loss by sleeping later than usual or napping during the day.

But if part of the reason you had a bad night was because your sleep drive wasn't high enough, this is like getting back on the road when you've just started filling the gas tank. In a short while, when you wake up, your tired tank will be empty again, and at that point, there's only enough time to partially fill it by bedtime. Without a full tired tank at night, you end up taking a long time to fall asleep, waking up throughout the night, and/or waking up too early.

Sleeping in after a bad night

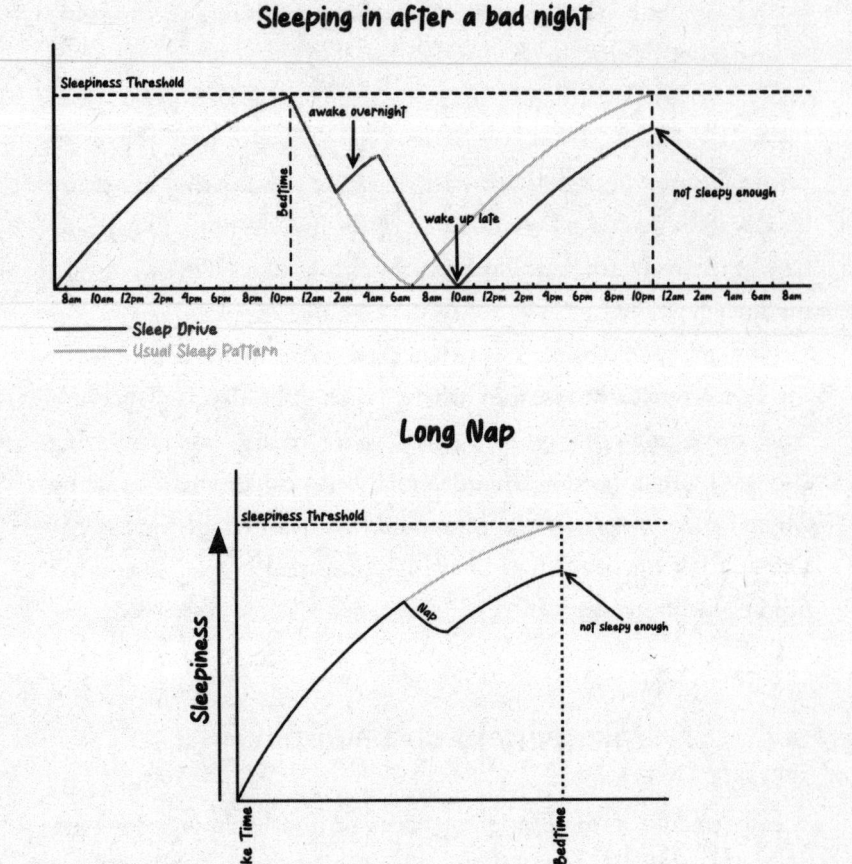

Long Nap

Insomniacs usually then perpetuate that cycle by sleeping in or nap-ping again to make up for *that* bad night. We're like a driver continu-ously pulling over to add small amounts of gas to the tank, instead of just waiting until the tank is full so we can get one long, efficient ride.

Early Bedtime

Finally, there's the tip that I would probably call the worst piece of advice to give an insomniac: if you want more sleep, go to bed earlier. My husband used to tell me this, my parents used to tell me this, even some sleep books advise this. The advice makes sense if you're sleep-deprived because you go to bed too late. But if your issue is that you go to bed but *can't* fall asleep or stay asleep, an early bedtime will only make matters worse. Just like in the scenario above, going to bed too early means going to bed before your tired tank is full, so you're going to bed before you're actually sleepy.

Sleepy vs. Tired vs. Fatigued

It's important to take a minute here to note what it means to be sleepy. Many of us use the words *tired* and *sleepy* interchangeably, but we also use *tired* to mean fatigued—and fatigue and sleepiness are not the same thing. Being sleepy or drowsy means you're struggling to stay awake. Some signs of sleepiness include heavy eyelids and difficulty holding your head up. That stranger next to you on the subway bobbing his head and maybe drooling on your shoulder—he's sleepy!

Fatigue, on the other hand, is when you're physically or mentally drained. A strenuous workout, a complicated task, or really any source of stress—including worries about sleep—can make you feel fatigued. Some signs of fatigue are heavy limbs, low energy, and an inability to concentrate. If this happens to you a lot for no apparent reason, tell your doctor, as there could be an underlying medical condition to blame. People who are fatigued often complain of feeling "tired," but when given the chance to nap, they can't fall asleep. And while it is possible to be both fatigued and sleepy, if you're just fatigued, you don't need sleep, you need rest.

I say this because like many insomniacs, I often made the mistake of going to bed when I felt fatigued, without realizing I wasn't actually sleepy. I would lie in bed with my eyes closed trying to will myself to sleep, but my sleep drive simply wasn't high enough. Soon the recognition that I wasn't asleep would start to frustrate me, and arousal would kick in. The result was almost always the same: I would fall asleep later than when I just went to bed at my usual bedtime.

And there lies the second part of the problem. When we sleep in, nap, or go to bed early, we deplete our sleep drive, which makes it hard to fall asleep or stay asleep. But that makes us frustrated—which leads to arousal. The higher our arousal, the higher our sleep drive needs to be to overpower it. And even though the root of the problem is that we're not sleepy enough, the stress of it all still makes us feel really tired. We then mistake that tiredness for sleepiness and respond . . . by trying to sleep in, nap, or go to bed early. This is how acute insomnia becomes chronic.

Insomnia

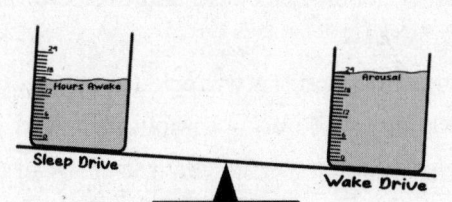

Chronic Insomnia

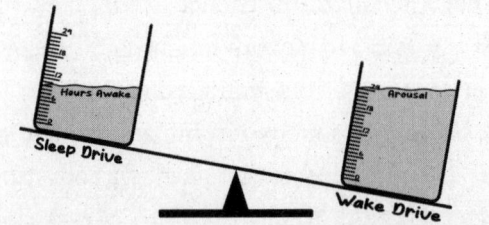

The good news is there are several ways to break this pattern, and interestingly enough our lack of sleep is the key ingredient to their success.

THE QUICK FIX:
INTENSIVE SLEEP RETRAINING

Intensive sleep retraining (ISR) is as close as you can get to a quick fix for chronic insomnia, but it will require you to skip an entire night of sleep. "Rip the Band-Aid off" types, this one's for you.

Accidentally discovered in the late 2000s, the treatment begins at a patient's usual bedtime and entails repeatedly giving them up to 25 minutes to fall asleep. But every time they do, they're woken up almost immediately. Researcher Dr. Hannah Scott tells me it's common in the beginning for patients to go all 25 minutes without falling asleep, in which case they're told to take a 5-minute break, then try again. But as the night ticks by, they start falling asleep faster and faster. Toward the end, insomniacs who report usually taking more than an hour to fall asleep are falling asleep within just 5 minutes and end up falling asleep quickly more than forty times over the course of the treatment.

Scott says that experience of falling asleep quickly over and over again gives patients "a lot more confidence that they're going to fall asleep more quickly after the lab study." And it appears they do. In the two weeks after intensive sleep retraining, patients in two studies reported falling asleep 24 to 30 minutes faster than they did before the treatment, and increasing their total amount of sleep by 34 to 60 minutes. Daytime fatigue and other impairments were also "significantly reduced" after treatment, and those treatment gains were largely maintained after six months.

"We think it's because it's extinguished that insomnia response, that learned response that they have when they're trying to sleep, and instead replaced it with a really strong response for falling asleep quickly," Scott tells me.

When I told my husband about this treatment, his response was "That sounds like pure torture!" But as someone who's had severe insomnia, all I could think was how badly I wished I'd known about this when I was struggling. Fixing insomnia by staying awake all night?! I was doing that anyway!

Yet even if you're well read on the topic of insomnia, you've probably never heard of intensive sleep retraining. Many sleep doctors don't even know about it! Scott believes that's because, in its original form, the treatment had to be done in a lab over the course of 24 hours, making it expensive and thus inaccessible.

But technology is quickly changing that. Thanks to apps like Sleep On Cue or devices like THIM, we can now do intensive sleep retraining at home—and in half the time. Rather than calculate sleep onset by monitoring patients under lab conditions, the new technology determines when you fall asleep through behavioral methods. Sleep On Cue, for example, periodically plays soft tones that you respond to by gently shaking your phone. Once you stop responding to the tones, the app concludes that you're asleep and wakes you up by vibrating the phone.

THIM, a wearable that goes on your finger, works in a similar way. It provides soft vibrations that you respond to by twitching your finger. Once you stop responding, THIM concludes you're asleep and delivers an intense vibration to wake you up.

Scott's research shows these methods are comparable to laboratory monitoring in predicting sleep onset, and she says a soon-to-be published study shows the at-home treatment results are also comparable to those from lab studies. "We've been able to successfully translate intensive sleep retraining to the home environment without impacting its efficacy . . . I'm pretty pumped about it!" she tells me.

I will warn that both Sleep On Cue and THIM's websites encourage users to do sleep retraining for just an hour or two after bedtime, then go to sleep as usual. In theory, doing this for a few nights in a row would mean trading one night of complete sleep deprivation for several nights of partial sleep deprivation, and trading immediate results for gradual results. But Scott says there's currently no clinical research to back this more gradual approach. If you want to try it that way, go for it. For a more clinically backed approach, try the protocol below based on Scott's research.

How-To: Intensive Sleep Retraining (ISR)

Warning: ISR will cause excessive sleepiness and may not be suitable for people who are sensitive to abrupt sleep changes—such as anyone with a history of seizures, migraines, or bipolar disorder. Do this only if you can avoid activities that would be dangerous while drowsy for a full day. For less risk of daytime sleepiness, try stimulus control or sleep compression instead, both described later in this chapter.

1. Get a clinically backed intensive sleep retraining app or device, like Sleep On Cue or THIM.
2. Choose a time when you can afford to be sleep-deprived two days in a row.
3. The night before starting the training, restrict your sleep to only five hours to ensure your sleep drive is high for the following night.
4. The night of retraining, starting at your usual bedtime, use your selected ISR device or app as instructed, preferably in your own bed.
5. Every time the device wakes you up, get out of bed, take a 5- to 10-minute break, then start again. It's best to leave the room during the break, but stick to quiet, relaxing activities and avoid bright light.
6. If you last the whole sleep opportunity without falling asleep, take a 5- to 10-minute break, then start again.
7. After forty sleep opportunities or twelve hours, whichever comes first, you're done.
8. Stay awake until at least two hours before your typical bedtime that night. No napping allowed! Avoid activities that are dangerous while drowsy, like driving.

(continued on next page)

9. Once you are within two hours of bedtime and feel very sleepy, go to bed for the night. Set your alarm for your target wake time (the time you want to wake up every day).
10. For best results, adhere to stimulus control rules for at least the next two weeks (see the next Fix for more on that).

The one area where ISR falls short is in helping people stay asleep. That might be part of the reason study participants who did both intensive sleep retraining and stimulus control, described below, saw even better results than those who did just one or the other. They also had much better compliance rates than those who only did stimulus control.

So intensive sleep retraining is a great way not only to see quick results in combating sleep onset insomnia but also to jump-start and ensure you'll stick with additional behavioral sleep therapies to combat sleep onset and sleep maintenance insomnia.

THE GRADUAL FIX:
STIMULUS CONTROL

Stimulus control is a common CBT-I technique that can either be used to maximize the results of intensive sleep retraining or can be used on its own for a more gradual approach to harnessing the power of your sleep drive and reestablishing your bed as a cue for sleep.

How-To: Stimulus Control

To implement stimulus control, just follow a few simple rules:

1. Use your bed for sleep and sex—that's it.
2. Establish a regular wake-up time. Stick to within an hour of that wake-up time even on your days off.

3. Go to bed only when sleepy (unless you're going there to have sex!).
4. If you're awake in bed long enough for it to bother you, get out of bed, do something relaxing, and try either of the following options:

- Return to bed when you feel sleepy.
- Predetermine how long you're going to stay out of bed—usually 30 minutes or an hour. If you get sleepy before then, try to stay awake until your selected time. No dozing on the couch!

Note: It's helpful to plan out some enjoyable, relaxing activities you can do ahead of time. Avoid anything that promotes wakefulness, like bright light. If you can't leave your bedroom, Dr. Jason Ellis suggests designating a special "wake zone" in the room for these activities. Shift workers, see chapter 14 for additional instructions.

5. Unless it's within 45 minutes of your wake time, don't decide to just start your day early. Even 30 minutes of additional sleep is worth the trip back to bed.
6. Preferably no napping. If you absolutely need to nap, try to do it at the same time every day for no more than 30 minutes.

After two weeks of stimulus control, if you're still struggling with insomnia, consider moving on to sleep restriction or sleep compression, both detailed below.

THE "SOUNDS WORSE THAN IT IS" FIX:
SLEEP RESTRICTION

Sleep restriction is the most widely known CBT-I technique and another good option for "rip the Band-Aid off" types.

The premise is simple. Restrict the amount of time you spend in bed until you start to fall asleep quickly and stay asleep. Then slowly increase your amount of time in bed until you're getting a sufficient amount of sleep but still sleeping efficiently.

My friend Brad still recalls when his sleep specialists first explained the concept to him. "They were like, 'This is going to sound weird, but you need to sleep less to sleep more,'" he said. At the time Brad was going to bed anywhere between 10:30 P.M. and 1:30 A.M., and waking up around 6:00 or 6:30 A.M., but he says a lot of that time wasn't actually spent sleeping. "I would be in bed and just be lying there super tired, but not asleep," he says.

Instead, Brad's specialists determined he should start going to bed around 12:30 A.M. and getting up around 5:30 A.M. Within two weeks he noticed he was sleeping more deeply and for longer blocks of time than he'd previously been able to. "This is what surprised me the most," he explains. "Even though the numbers in terms of 'Oh, you need to sleep for nine hours a night' weren't there, I just felt so much better."

Over time, Brad's specialists then expanded his sleep window by fifteen minutes a week. Now he says he sleeps every night from roughly midnight to 6:45 A.M. "And I feel amazing," he adds.

Sleep restriction is ideally done under the guidance of a trained CBT-I therapist, like Brad's, who will tell you exactly what times to get into and out of bed. But studies have shown it can be an effective self-help tool as well, so Dr. S. Justin Thomas and Dr. Daniel Erichsen helped me create the user-friendly guide below. And while the term *sleep restriction* sounds scary, the real goal is not to restrict your sleep, but rather to consolidate it.

How-To: Sleep Restriction

Warning: Sleep restriction can cause daytime sleepiness and may not be suitable for people who are sensitive to abrupt sleep changes—such as anyone with a history of seizures, migraine, or bipolar disorder. Do this only if you can avoid activities that would be dangerous while drowsy, at least for the first few days. For less risk of daytime sleepiness, try stimulus control or sleep compression, also described in this chapter, instead.

1. Use the tools from chapter 4 and/or a week's worth of sleep diary entries to estimate how much sleep you usually get between your bedtime and your wake time. This does not have to be exact. (*Note:* Sleep trackers are not recommended for this.)
2. Restrict your allowed time in bed to only the amount of time you usually spend asleep. If you struggle to fall asleep, do this by sliding your bedtime later. If you struggle to stay asleep, slide your wake time earlier. If you struggle to fall asleep and stay asleep, make bedtime later and wake time earlier.

   - For example, if you usually spend 8 hours in bed but sleep for only 6 of those hours, you'll need to cut 2 hours out of your sleep window. You can do this by going to bed 2 hours later, waking up 2 hours earlier, or going to bed 1 hour later and waking 1 hour earlier.
   - Your sleep window should be at least 5.5 hours. Don't restrict more than that even if you think you sleep less.
   - You can opt to add an extra 30 minutes to your sleep window as a buffer.

3. Don't go to bed until your new bedtime or later, and don't go to bed until you feel sleepy.
4. If at any point you're awake in bed long enough for it to bother you, get out of bed, do something enjoyable and relaxing, and return to bed when you feel sleepy.
5. Get out of bed at your designated wake time or earlier. No hitting the snooze bar, no sleeping in.
6. No napping or dozing allowed! You cannot sleep at all outside your designated sleep window.
7. Fight the urge to cheat or quit. It'll become harder to stay awake until your bedtime, but in a few days you'll start falling asleep faster, sleeping more deeply, and staying asleep longer—your body is making up for sleep *quantity* by improving sleep *quality*.
8. Once you're sleeping through the night, or waking only briefly, and are satisfied with how long it takes you to fall asleep, expand your sleep window by 15 minutes every week until you feel you're getting enough sleep but are still sleeping efficiently.

   - The general guideline for good sleep efficiency is when you spend 85 to 90 percent of your time in bed asleep, but don't get too caught up in doing the math—the exact number doesn't matter.

9. If you start to have trouble falling asleep or staying asleep again, reverse course. This may be a sign that you have exceeded the amount of time you should be spending in bed.

Digital Sleep Restriction

For sleep restriction with a bit more guidance, check out the digital CBT-I options mentioned in chapter 2. The CBT-i Coach app, for example, will tell you specific times to go to bed and wake up based on your sleep diary entries in the app—and it's free!

THE "EASE INTO IT" FIX:
SLEEP COMPRESSION

If the thought of doing sleep restriction scares the crap out of you, you might want to try sleep compression instead. Like sleep restriction, sleep compression works to reduce your awake time in bed, but instead of abruptly cutting your sleep window down, then gradually increasing it, you reach your goal by gradually decreasing time in bed. If you're not a "rip the Band-Aid off" type, this one's for you!

Dr. S. Justin Thomas, director of the University of Alabama at Birmingham Behavioral Sleep Medicine Clinic, tells me he prefers sleep compression for patients who might be sensitive to abrupt changes in their sleep schedule. He also says there's less risk of over-restricting time in bed, so less risk of daytime sleepiness. I also like it because it requires less math!

But despite its benefits, in all the books and articles I've read on insomnia, sleep compression didn't get a single mention outside of academic textbooks. It makes me wonder how many people may be avoiding CBT-I entirely because they fear sleep restriction and don't realize there are other options. The guide below was put together with the help of Dr. S. Justin Thomas and Dr. Daniel Erichsen.

How-To: Sleep Compression

1. Decide how quickly you want to reduce or "compress" your sleep window. There are no set rules, but Dr. Thomas says a very general guideline is 15 to 30 minutes per week. Faster compressions bring faster results but also a higher risk of daytime impairment.
2. If you struggle to fall asleep, compress your sleep window by sliding your bedtime later. If you struggle to stay asleep, slide your wake time earlier. If you struggle to fall asleep and stay asleep, make your bedtime later and your wake time earlier.

    -   For example, if you're compressing 30 minutes a week, you can go to bed 30 minutes later, wake up 30 minutes earlier, or go to bed 15 minutes later and wake up 15 minutes earlier each week.

3. Don't go to bed until your new bedtime or later, and don't go to bed until you feel sleepy.
4. If at any point you're awake in bed long enough for it to bother you, get out of bed, do something enjoyable and relaxing, and return to bed when you feel sleepy.
5. Get out of bed at your designated wake time or earlier. No hitting the snooze bar, no sleeping in.
6. No napping or dozing allowed! You cannot sleep at all outside your designated sleep window.
7. Keep compressing until you are sleeping through the night, or waking only briefly, and are satisfied with how long it takes you to fall asleep.

    -   The general guideline for good sleep efficiency is when you spend 85 to 90 percent of your time in bed asleep, but don't get too caught up in doing the math—the exact number doesn't matter.
    -   If your sleep efficiency starts to decrease again, pick up where you left off and resume compressing.
    -   Don't compress beyond 5.5 hours of total time in bed. If you hit this and you still don't think you're sleeping efficiently, see a sleep specialist.
    -   If after a few days of sleeping efficiently you feel sleepy during the day, slowly increase your sleep window. This could be an indication that you need more sleep. If that doesn't help, contact a professional.

What I Did

When I was battling my insomnia, I hadn't heard of sleep compression or stimulus control. So, given my odd schedule, I decided to try my own modified version of sleep restriction. Unbeknownst to me, this ended up incorporating some elements of all three.

At the time, not only was I working nocturnal hours, but I could get home from work as early as 5:00 A.M. or as late as 9:00 A.M., and then on occasion I'd get called back for extra shoots in the late morning, afternoon, or evening. So rather than setting a wake time and working backward, as is commonly suggested, I did things the other way around and started with my bedtime instead.

Dr. Stern emphasized that consistency was more important than time of day. So, despite the fact that it was easier and more convenient for me to fall asleep at 5:00 A.M. than 9:00 A.M., I set 9:00 A.M. as my earliest allowed bedtime, since I could do that almost every day.

I also spoke to my boss about my sleep issues and my schedule. Together we established that from roughly 9:00 A.M. to 3:00 P.M., I would be considered unavailable for work, barring breaking news. This way, even on my busiest days, I could still have roughly six hours in bed.

Finally, I set my wake time (provided I didn't get called into work sooner) as 5:00 P.M.—eight hours after my allowed bedtime. This was far more than my usual amount of sleep, but it was still significantly less than the twelve hours I was sometimes spending in bed. It also allowed me to be more relaxed on the days I got home after nine, because I knew I had enough time to unwind and still get a good amount of sleep in before I had to get up. I also figured I could always restrict further if I needed to.

So my sleep restriction/compression rules started off like this:

1. No going to bed before 9:00 A.M.
2. No going to bed unless sleepy
3. No napping

4. No staying in bed past 5:00 P.M. (eight hours after allowed bedtime)

At first I was all over the place. On late workdays I would come home wired and wouldn't feel sleepy until at least 10:00 A.M. When I got home closer to 5:00 A.M., I found it hard to stay up until nine. This was especially tough on weekends, when I spent the night in a quiet apartment with a sleeping husband, rather than in a bustling studio full of other awake people. I would also often wake up prematurely and be up for a while. If I was able to fall back asleep, it was a serious struggle to then force myself out of bed when the alarm went off at 5:00 P.M.

But I stuck with it. After a week or two my sleep started to improve and I compressed my sleep window more, sliding my allowed bedtime to 9:30 A.M. and my wake time to 4:30 P.M. I was falling asleep faster and faster and staying asleep longer and longer. I also started finding it easier to fall back asleep if I woke up prematurely. And those wake-ups became less and less frequent.

Three weeks later I retook my sleep structure test and Dr. Stern said I was getting 6.5 hours with a nearly normal ratio of light sleep to deep sleep. That grew to an estimated 7 to 8 hours of sleep, and eventually settled around 6.5 to 7 hours, which still feels like the right ballpark for me.

Pro Tip: Reverse Curfew

When setting up your own sleep schedule don't underestimate the power of what I call a reverse curfew—aka banning yourself from going to bed before a certain time. It may sound counterintuitive, but by challenging yourself to stay awake rather than forcing yourself to fall asleep you can alleviate some of the performance anxiety that comes with insomnia, in addition to increasing your sleep drive. Just make sure you're still doing relatively sleep-friendly activities. It will not help you to blow past your bedtime by playing a fast-paced video game or endlessly scrolling through Instagram.

THE BONUS FIX:
EXERCISE

Aside from staying awake, the only other known way to increase adenosine is to exercise. So a good workout won't just make you tired—it can actually make you sleepy.

WWE star Kofi Kingston, a friend of mine from college, credits exercise with part of the reason he can sleep despite his crazy travel schedule. "I feel strange if I don't exercise," he tells me. "I've been working out since college consistently . . . I'd be surprised if that didn't help you fall asleep as easily as I do."

Jason Karp also credits exercise with helping him get his sleep back on track. "I found that if I exercised aggressively to the point of exhaustion, it actually allowed me to sleep longer," he says. "So I started reincorporating exercise . . . at least an hour a day."

Granted, I realize most of us are probably not going to work out as vigorously or consistently as Kofi and Jason do, but unfortunately, most people suffering from insomnia do the complete opposite. We forgo our usual physical activities to spend more time in bed, trying to recover lost sleep. Once we finally give up and get out of bed, we're still tired and less inclined to be physically active. This lack of exercise then weakens our sleep drive, which makes it harder for us to fall asleep or stay asleep and feeds our insomnia cycle.

So as hard as it may seem, during times of the day you want to be awake, get your body moving in any way that seems feasible. Besides making you feel more alert in the moment, this can also help ease anxiety and give you an extra boost of sleepiness at bedtime. (See chapter 12 for more on how exercise can affect sleep.)

PART 3

CIRCADIAN RHYTHM VS. SCHEDULE

If sleep drive increases the longer we're awake, you'd expect our energy to steadily decrease all day. But instead, we experience dips in our energy at certain times and then "catch a second wind." So what's up? Enter circadian rhythm.

Circadian rhythm is a biological clock that, along with sleep drive, controls our sleep/wake cycle. While our sleep drive steadily increases if we're awake and decreases if we're asleep, circadian rhythm dips and rises throughout the day, making us feel more or less awake at certain times—regardless of whether or not we've slept. It's like a wake drive on autopilot. So while things like stress, excitement, and relaxation all affect our arousal levels, our circadian rhythm does too.

Circadian rhythm varies from person to person, but generally it rises throughout the morning, takes a dip in the afternoon (hence the midday slump), then rises again in the evening before diving for the night. When paired against our sleep drive it looks something like this example of someone who sleeps from 11:00 P.M. to 7:00 A.M.

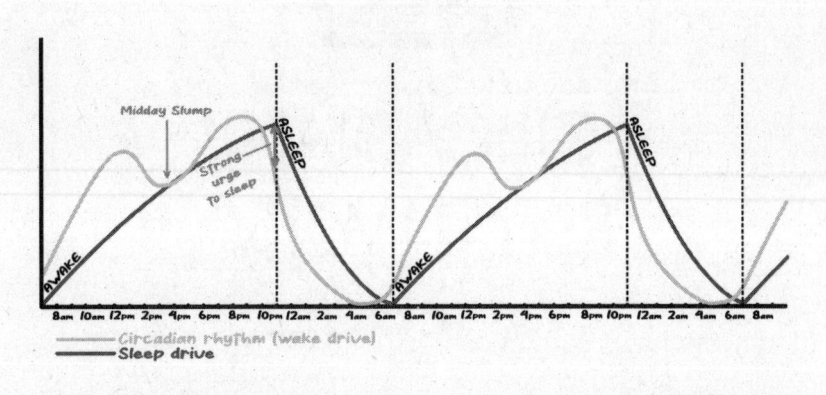

The ideal time to go to bed is when our circadian rhythm starts taking its big nightly dive. If we've been awake all day, our sleep drive will be high. Provided we're reasonably relaxed, that high sleep drive plus our dropping circadian wake drive makes it easy to fall asleep. Then while we sleep, our sleep drive diminishes, but our circadian wake drive drops too, keeping us asleep. After bottoming out in the overnight hours, our circadian wake drive rises again in the morning, waking us up and giving us increasing energy. Thanks to all that sleep we got, our sleep drive is eliminated, and we're ready to face the day.

Sounds great, right? It is . . . when it works that way. But when your schedule and circadian rhythm are out of sync, it can wreak havoc on your sleep and general well-being. Most of you will have already experienced this in the form of jet lag. While you want to sleep and wake according to the time zone you're in, your circadian rhythm is still set to your old time zone. So your wake drive is high when you're trying to sleep, and low when you're trying to wake up.

The result can be daytime fatigue, sleepiness, inability to sleep, stomach issues, and just generally feeling like crap.

In my case, this was my everyday existence—for years. Day after day, I would wake up for my bizarre work schedule at a time my circadian wake drive was really low. Then when I got home, I would try to sleep when my circadian wake drive was really high. Because of that, I wasn't able to fall asleep for a long time, which meant when the alarm clock went off again, I had slept only a few hours. So not only was I battling a low wake drive again due to the time of day, but due to my lack of sleep now my sleep drive was high too. It's hard to express how difficult it is to get out of bed and get through the day when both of these forces are working against you. Your limbs feel heavy, like you're walking through quicksand. Once your circadian rhythm starts to rise, the heaviness starts to dissipate, but your high sleep drive still leaves you feeling foggy, achy, tired, and any number of other symptoms.

To make matters worse, I then developed conditioned arousal (see chapter 3) from all that time I spent awake and frustrated in bed, and just like that, I was unknowingly facing a one-two punch: a circadian rhythm disorder *and* insomnia.

When I went searching for answers, the most common one I found was to quit my job. But quitting a job is a huge change that can carry major consequences. And I loved my job. Also, as you'll learn in the next few chapters, you don't have to work bizarre hours to suffer from circadian rhythm issues. This isn't just a night shift problem—which makes it even less realistic that everyone whose schedule is off is just going to quit their job for better sleep.

Luckily, there is another way. While circadian rhythm is often portrayed as an immovable obstacle, we do eventually adjust to jet lag. Why? Because our circadian rhythm takes cues from when we eat, when we sleep, when we're active, and most of all, when we see light and dark, and it resets accordingly. We can use these same cues to not only speed up jet lag recovery but also to help with every other circadian disorder as well.

CHAPTER 6

Chronotypes

WHAT TIME YOUR CIRCADIAN RHYTHM hits its daily highs and lows is what determines whether you're naturally inclined to fall asleep and wake up early or fall asleep and wake up late—aka your chronotype. People often split chronotypes into two categories—night owls and early birds—and view them as a choice or a reflection of your character, as if being a morning person means you're more responsible or disciplined than someone who isn't. But your chronotype is actually part of your biology.

Chronotypes are also part of a spectrum that sleep experts generally divide into at least three categories, not two. Where you land on that spectrum may have a lot to do with your sleep problems.

Chronotype 1:
Early Bird/Morning Type

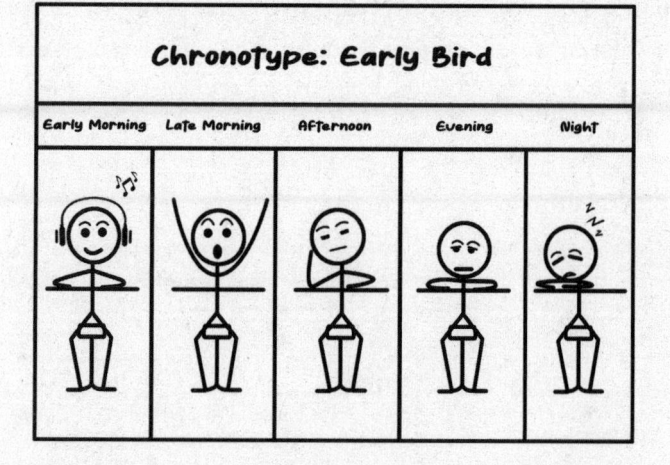

Chronotype: Early Bird

| Early Morning | Late Morning | Afternoon | Evening | Night |

Early birds or morning types are people who naturally wake up early, full of energy, and get tired early in the evening. This group is also sometimes called larks.

Chronotype 2:
Hummingbird/Intermediate Type

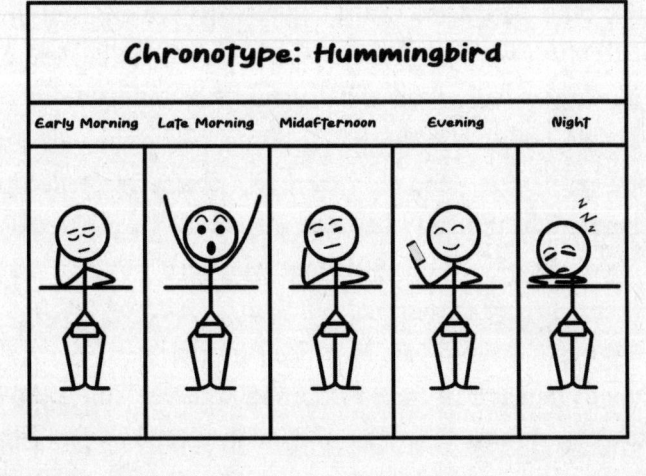

Hummingbirds or intermediate types feel alert by midmorning and sleepy by mid- to late evening. If this sounds normal to you, it's because, according to Dr. Michael Breus, about 50 percent of the population falls into this category. This group is also sometimes referred to as *neither,* as in neither morning nor evening oriented.

Chronotype 3:
Night Owl/Evening Type

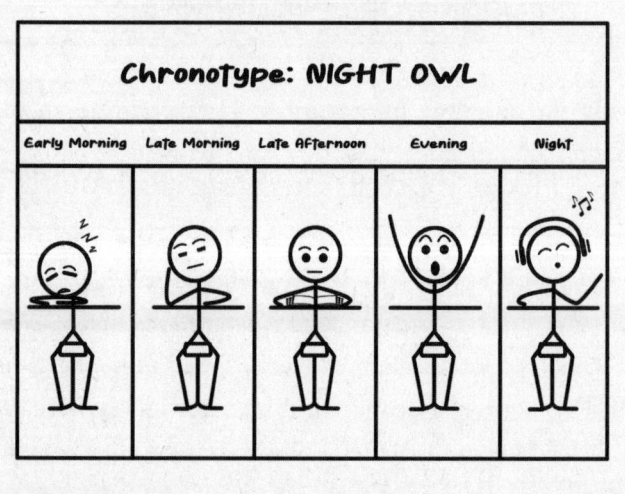

Night owls or evening types often have the hardest time of all three chronotypes working typical hours. Breus says this group doesn't feel sleepy until roughly midnight or later, and has a hard time waking up before nine A.M. They feel most alert in the evening, when most others are winding down.

As someone who was always the "last man standing" after any social event, I've been called a night owl more times than I can count. The term is *very* familiar to me. But I always thought being a night owl just meant I *liked* being up late. I had no idea it meant that I was *naturally* programmed to be up late, and I certainly had no idea that it was my chronotype.

Still, while chronotypes are rarely mentioned in your average listicle of sleep tips, identifying your chronotype can be a huge help in determining if your circadian rhythm is contributing to your sleep difficulties and how you can best deal with that.

THE FOR NOW FIX:
CHRONOTYPE QUESTIONNAIRE

Currently the only way to measure your exact circadian rhythm is through blood or saliva tests that can't be done at home, something circadian researchers hope to change in the coming years. The next best option is the Munich Chronotype Questionnaire (MCTQ), which has been shown in studies to provide a very accurate estimate. But the questionnaire is pretty long and tallying the results involves a lot of math . . . bleck. Thankfully, the creator of the MCTQ, Dr. Till Roenneberg from Ludwig-Maximilian University, helped me put together a simple four-part questionnaire to use instead.

Roenneberg says the quick questionnaire won't provide the kind of accuracy needed for scientific studies, and the categories in the chart below can differ based on geographical location and culture (I think they skew a bit early compared to typical American wake-up times), but it should still be sufficient to offer a general assessment of how morning or evening oriented you are, which will help you apply the rest of the tools in this part of the book.

How-To: Quick Chronotype Questionnaire

When answering the following questions, imagine a staycation scenario in which you have your home completely to yourself for a few days to settle into sleeping and waking with your body's natural rhythm. All other members of your household—including pets—are out of the house, and you have no obligations, interruptions, or sleep obstacles of any kind.

1. What time do you think you would naturally fall sleep? (*Note:* This is not what time you'd go to bed, it's what time you'd actually fall asleep.)
2. What time do you think you would naturally wake up? (*Note:* This is without an alarm clock.)
3. What's the midpoint between your natural sleep time and your natural wake time? (For example, if you estimate you'd sleep from midnight to 8:00 A.M., the midpoint would be 4:00 A.M.)
4. Use the table below to connect your midpoint to your chronotype:

MIDPOINT OF UNRESTRICTED SLEEP	CHRONOTYPE
11 p.m. – 1:30 a.m.	Extremely Early
1:30 a.m. – 2:30 a.m.	Moderately Early
2:30 a.m. – 3:30 a.m.	Slightly Early
3:30 a.m. – 5 a.m.	Intermediate
5 a.m. – 6 a.m.	Slightly Late
6 a.m. – 7 a.m.	Moderately Late
7 a.m. – 11:30 a.m.	Extremely Late

Based on MSF in the MCTQ database July 2017

CHAPTER 7

Scheduling

CHRONOTYPES ARE BELIEVED TO BE influenced by genetics and age—two things we can't control. Most of us are early birds as babies, night owls as teens, and we tend to shift earlier again in our later years. But other than get older, there's nothing we can do to change our chronotype, yet you would never know that from general expectations about how we should schedule our lives. We're constantly hearing old sayings like "You snooze, you lose," "The early bird gets the worm," and "Early to bed and early to rise, makes a man healthy, wealthy, and wise." And the advice goes beyond adages. How many articles have you seen about how super successful people are early risers?

There's no shortage of write-ups on how Apple CEO Tim Cook wakes up at 3:45 A.M. or former PepsiCo CEO Indra Nooyi wakes up at 4:00 A.M. Dwayne "the Rock" Johnson is so notorious for waking up early, he created an alarm clock app to help others do the same (the app is hilarious, by the way). And Mark Wahlberg, who might be the king of early risers, made headlines when he revealed he wakes up at 2:30 A.M. The overwhelming message is that to be successful (and/or to have washboard abs), you too must rise before the sun. But this approach completely disregards chronotypes.

Common sleep advice often does the same. When I was a teen, my parents always told me how much better off I would be if I woke up early to finish my studies, rather than staying up late. That might have been true . . . for them. But as a night owl teen, I can tell you that the few times I tried waking up early to study, it did *not* go well. And I always managed to get good grades despite (or maybe even because of) my late-night study habits.

Shift Workers in Disguise

Standard work schedules also disregard chronotypes. We always hear about the difficulties of shift work, which is often defined as working "abnormal" hours like a night or early morning shift. But whether a schedule is normal for you depends on your chronotype.

WWE star Kofi Kingston tells me his usual schedule of traveling and putting on wrestling shows at night means he can't get to bed until around 2:00 A.M., but as a night owl, Kofi sleeps just fine on that schedule. "When I'm on the road, I can get a good seven, eight hours. Then I'll wake up and go to the gym and wash, rinse, repeat for the next four days," he tells me. Interestingly, it's when Kofi's not working that his sleep takes a hit, because he still goes to bed around 2:00 A.M., but at home his kids wake him up around seven-thirty. "I have a lot of energy . . . but in the mornings, I'm just kind of groggy," he tells me.

Just as Kofi does well on a late schedule, early birds on the early morning shift would be very much in line with their circadian rhythm. But give a night owl "normal" hours, and that 6:00 or 7:00 A.M. alarm is likely forcing them to wake up before they've had enough sleep and before their circadian wake drive is high enough to help them feel awake—a double whammy of sleepiness that can last well into the morning. Because of this, night owls often struggle with an unfair perception of being lazy. In reality, they're just shift workers in disguise. Those who try to avoid this by going to bed too early can also end up with insomnia (see part 2 for more on that).

When my former co-anchor Kendis Gibson started working mornings at CNN in Atlanta, his wake-up time was 4:30 A.M. While that's early, it's not what we would traditionally consider shift work. But as a night owl, Kendis would only naturally start feeling sleepy around midnight, making it nearly impossible for him to get enough sleep. "And when you're living in the South, obviously, it gets darker later. It was just tough to turn myself down," he tells me. Left to his own devices, Kendis also wakes up around 9:00 A.M. So with a 4:30 wake-up call, he was essentially jet-lagged by nearly five hours—every single day. Which looks something like this:

Circadian Rhythm 5 Hours Behind Sleep Schedule

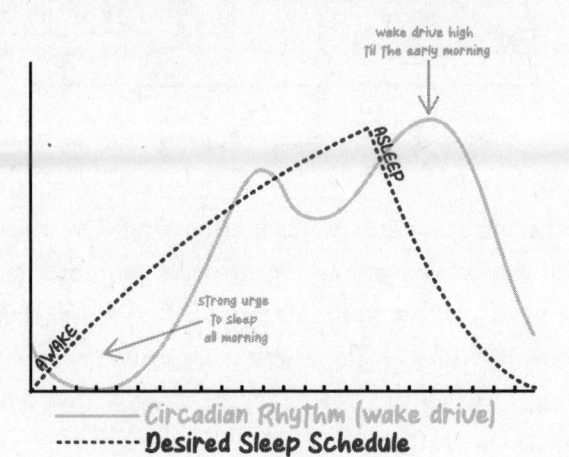

Now at MSNBC, Kendis is back to anchoring early mornings on weekends. He says having to wake up early twice a week is easier than doing it five days a week, but he still relies on Ambien to get enough sleep on those days.

An early bird on the evening shift could have an equally hard time. They'll be stuck at work after their wake drive has dropped and likely be forced to go to bed much later than their natural bedtime. Then their circadian rhythm will still force them awake in the early morning hours, leaving them sleep-deprived. The next evening they'll have to struggle through both a low wake drive *and* a high sleep drive.

Circadian Rhythm 5 Hours Ahead of Sleep Schedule

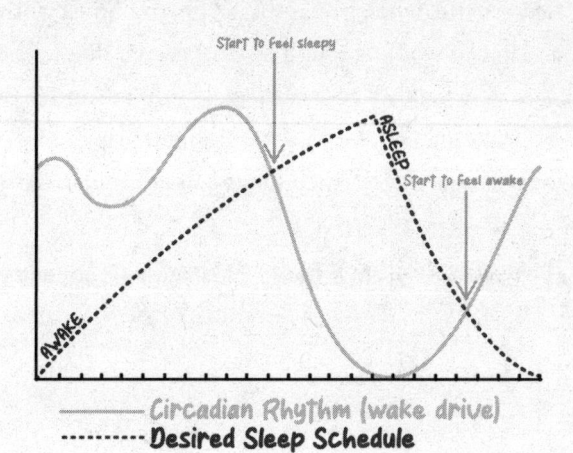

Start to feel sleepy

ASLEEP

Start to feel awake

AWAKE

——— Circadian Rhythm (wake drive)
·········· Desired Sleep Schedule

My mother, who says she's most alert from 6:00 A.M. to 2:00 P.M., experienced this while working for our local church. Most of the time she worked 10:00 A.M. to 2:00 P.M., but once a week her shift was 3:00 P.M. to 9:00 P.M. She describes those days as "hoooooooorrible," saying, "I would struggle, struggle, struggle, to keep awake, really struggle."

Mom says the day was easier if she had a lot of visitors, but if she was stuck with mostly paperwork to do, she was in trouble. "Being at the desk . . . was hard, very hard for me. I would have to stand up and walk around a little bit and then come back to whatever I was doing," she explains. "It took me much longer to do stuff than in my regular working hours." Mom says she was also much more prone to mistakes during her evening shift, and always had to review her work once she was back to her regular hours.

Luckily, Mom did this late shift only once a week and still made it home in time for her usual bedtime. We also lived close enough to the church that she could walk home rather than drive. But Mom's other job, being a court interpreter, would occasionally require her to drive home from a late case. "I remember coming from court around five-thirty . . . It was a struggle for me to keep my concentration," she says.

So not only do these scenarios carry health consequences but they can also be outright dangerous for those who need to be alert to do their jobs safely and for those who have to drive before or after their shift.

Social Jet Lag

Unlike my mother, most of us consider our weekday alarm to be an early wake-up call, and come the weekend, we look forward to sleeping in. Knowing we don't have to wake up early, we also tend to stay up later. The problem is our body, eager to get back to its natural rhythm, quickly adjusts to those weekend hours. When Sunday bedtime hits, we're wide awake with the "Sunday scaries." Welcome to social jet lag.

We usually readjust to our weekday schedule after a few days . . . just in time to do it all over again the following weekend.

Insomnia

Insomniacs trying to get their sleep back on track often make the same mistakes as those with social jet lag. We sleep in if we have a bad night, hoping to make up for our sleep debt. But Dr. Jason Ong says this is a classic way insomniacs "shoot themselves in the foot," because doing so not only depletes our sleep drive, it paves the way for another late night. If we do this enough, we confuse our biological clock into thinking we're *supposed* to be going to bed later and waking up later *going forward*. Ong calls this the "spiral into chronic insomnia."

Of course, most of us will still be forced into schedules that aren't perfect for our circadian rhythm, because of jobs, babies—life. The next few chapters will cover how to manipulate your circadian rhythm to better suit your schedule. But the bigger the difference is between your circadian rhythm and your sleep schedule, the more difficult it will be to get them to work together. So to the extent you can, use the recommendations below to help your schedule work with you, rather than against you.

THE STARTING POINT FIX:
CONSIDER CHRONOTYPE

It may be trendy to be an early riser, and yes, many high-powered executives and celebrities seem to achieve great success with their predawn morning routines #4amclub. But you know who else has achieved great success? Reddit founder Alexis Ohanian, who reportedly "tries" to be up by 10:00 A.M. and doesn't go to bed until around 2:00 A.M. Tesla and SpaceX founder Elon Musk says he goes to bed at roughly 1:00 A.M. and sleeps until seven. Facebook CEO Mark Zuckerberg, a notorious night owl, once said he sleeps until 8:00 A.M., and that was after saying his daughter made him more of a morning person. Grammy winner Pharrell Williams reportedly goes to bed between midnight and 2:00 A.M. and wakes up at nine. And, as I already mentioned, WWE star Kofi Kingston doesn't go to bed until 2:00 A.M., even on his days off.

Kofi tells me the main reason he goes to bed so late when he's not working is that he waits until his kids go to bed to get his errands and workout done. As someone who spends a lot of time on the road, Kofi says maximizing family time is his top priority. "Just being in the presence of my family brings me the most joy," he tells me.

Of course Kofi could instead wake up extra early to get his stuff done before his kids wake up, but he tells me, "It undoubtedly works better for me to work out late, as I tend to have more energy at night." Considering his long list of accolades, including 2019 WWE Champion, the late nights seem to be working for him.

So to the extent you can control your schedule, respect your chronotype. If you're a natural early riser, enjoy that sunrise. But if you're an evening type, don't front-load your morning with activities you can do later in the day. Just because people don't share as many Instagram pics of their late-night productivity doesn't mean it's not happening. And just because Mark Walhberg wakes up at 2:30 A.M. doesn't mean you have to!

For any employers reading this, consider chronotypes when creating employee schedules too. If your business needs everybody in by nine A.M. to function, by all means make that your start time. But if your shift hours exist simply because "that's the way we've always done it," it may be time for an update. In the words of shift work sleep consultant Carolyn Schur, "we are missing out on the contributions and the skills and the creativity of night owl types, because we're forcing them to do it nine to four" . . . or in many cases eight to six. (See more on shift work in chapter 14.)

THE TRIED AND TRUE FIX:
CONSISTENT WAKE-UP TIME

Ask a sleep expert for tips to promote sleep health, and there's a good chance one of the first answers you'll get is "wake up at the same time every day." One reason for this is that most people's circadian rhythm is actually slightly longer than twenty-four hours, meaning our sleep and wake times have a natural inclination to drift later and later. As Dr. Jason Ong explains, "Getting up at the same time—and ideally getting exposed to light—is really what's most important to keep it on a twenty-four-hour cycle." Stick to this schedule and Ong says your brain starts to set its clock to that clear, consistent wake-up time and morning light. Eventually you start waking without the alarm clock and feeling sleepy at the same time every night.

The other thing about wake time: it's the part we can control. We can't dictate exactly when we fall asleep, but thanks to alarm clocks, we can ensure we wake up by a certain time. The exception to this is extreme morning types, who fall asleep and wake up too early. Since you can't force yourself to wake up later, you'll want to focus on delaying your bedtime and using the other techniques in the next few chapters to push your circadian rhythm later too.

But as with most sleep tips, your schedule doesn't have to be perfect, just try to keep things reasonably consistent. For those who can't because of rotating shift work, for example, see chapter 14 for more on how to establish a compromise circadian position.

THE ROTATING FIX:
MOVE CLOCKWISE

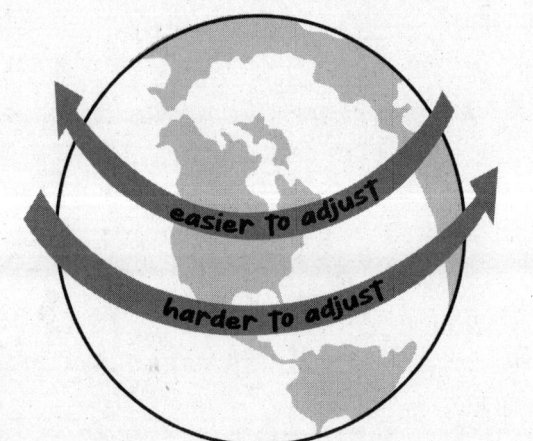

Unless you're an extreme morning type, it is easier to delay than advance circadian rhythms. So if you're planning a multi-stop trip, plan it so you're moving east to west. And if you're a rotating shift worker, try to arrange your schedule so it starts with your earliest shift and then progressively moves later. More on this in chapter 14.

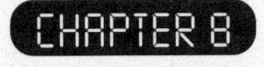

Light/Dark Contrast

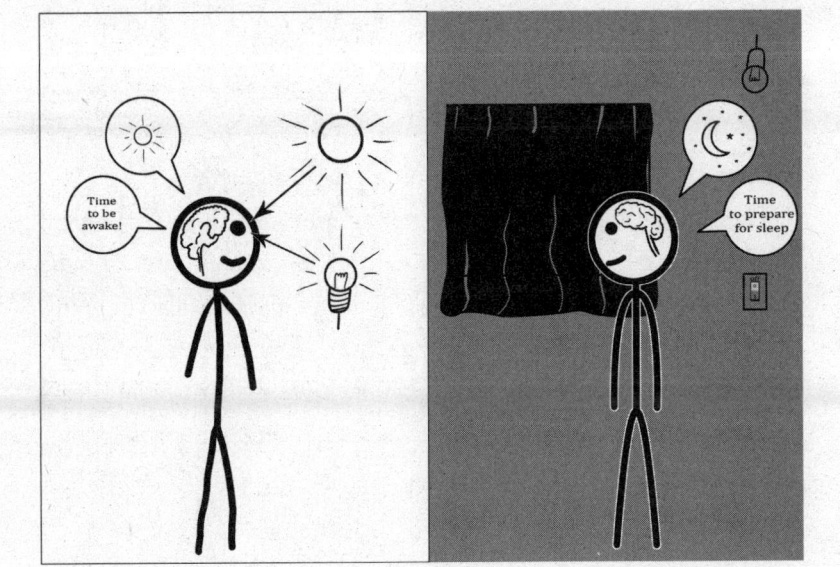

THE MOST POWERFUL CUES FOR your circadian rhythm are light and dark. When we see darkness, our brain releases a hormone called melatonin, which tells our body it's time to sleep. When we see bright light, especially sunlight, melatonin is suppressed and our cortisol levels rise, helping us to feel awake. In a way, we're solar powered.

We most commonly hear this discussed in the context of how blue light from screens is ruining our sleep. But all the talk about screens often misses all the other light sources impacting our circadian rhythm, which are arguably more significant and easier to avoid. It also misses the other way we can limit the effects of evening light—getting more light during the day.

That's because circadian cues are all about contrast. The bigger the contrast between how much light we get during the day versus how much we get at night, the clearer it is to our circadian rhythm when we're meant to be awake and when we're meant to be sleeping.

Unfortunately for our circadian rhythm, most humans no longer spend their days outside getting up to 100,000 lux of brightness from the sun. Instead, most of us spend the majority of our day indoors, where we're lucky if we get 500 lux of light. As Dr. Satchin Panda writes in his book *The Circadian Code*, "If the only time you can recall seeing the sky is when you are driving to or from work, chances are you are not getting enough natural daylight."

Then at the end of our day, we complicate things further by flooding our environments with roughly the same amount of light we get at the office. So as the day begins and ends, instead of going from bright light to no light, we go from dim light to dim light. This hinders our circadian clock's ability to tell what time it is and has a number of negative consequences, including trouble sleeping.

THE DARKNESS FIX:
THE FOUR D'S

If you struggle to fall asleep at night, one of the best things you can do for your circadian rhythm is reduce the amount of light you're exposed to in the four to five hours before you go to bed. This allows your brain to register that it's nighttime and sets the stage for that much-needed circadian dive.

How dim is dim enough? The unsatisfying answer is, it depends. A 2019 study on how much evening light it takes to cause a 50 percent drop in melatonin found results ranging from just 6 lux, in the most sensitive participant, to 350 lux in the least sensitive, after five hours of exposure. But most participants experienced that drop around 25 lux. Now consider that most residential rooms are lit anywhere from 100 to 500 lux, and you can understand why we might have trouble sleeping at night.

Of course most of us don't walk around with a lux meter, so a much easier solution is to just eliminate unnecessary light by remembering the Four D's: *dimness, distance, duration, direction.* Lowering brightness, being farther away from a light, facing it away from your eyes, and cutting the amount of time you're exposed to it all help to reduce overall exposure.

Once I started paying attention to the Four D's, I realized my husband and I had some fixable light habits. We regularly turned on lights we didn't need, left them on after we no longer needed them, and kept them on way brighter than we needed, despite having dimmer switches. Just addressing those issues has not only helped my sleep and the environment, it's also been great for our electric bill.

For those who struggle with waking up too early, you'll want to instead limit your light exposure when you wake up. This sends your brain the message that it's still nighttime, not wake-up time.

Lamps

As a former overnight shifter and someone who still occasionally works late hours, I made lighting changes in my office too. Since the overheads there are non-dimmable fluorescents, I have them on early in the day. But later in the day I turn them off in favor of some dimmable lamps. Anything to warm the lighting color and reduce the amount of light hitting the eye.

No Dimmer? No Problem

Technology is making dimming lights easier than ever with bulbs you can now dim without a dimmer switch. Just turn them on, off, and back on again, to toggle between different brightness levels. Some change color tone as well.

Night-Lights

For a super-affordable option, use a standard night-light, as I did in my bathroom. Now, come evening time, I no longer need to turn on the super-bright overhead light. I just flick on the night-light and I have a relaxing, sleep-friendly environment for brushing my teeth, bathing, or taking the occasional middle-of-the-night bathroom break.

Sunglasses

If that all seems like too much work, you can go with the lowest tech option of all: sunglasses. In his book *The Circadian Code,* Dr. Satchin Panda points out that sunglasses can reduce the amount of light reaching the eye by seven- to fifteenfold! And sure, you might look a little ridiculous wearing sunglasses at night, but just add an earpiece and you can pretend you're in the Secret Service.

THE LIGHT FIX:
BRIGHT LIGHT THERAPY

Limiting light exposure hours before bed isn't an option for everyone, and either way, the more light contrast between your sleep time and wake time, the better. Enter bright light therapy.

Common advice dictates we get bright light first thing in the morning to help our sleep. This is good advice for most, but again it depends on what you're hoping to accomplish. Bright light around our wake time helps us phase advance our circadian clock, encouraging us to fall asleep and wake up earlier. Bright light around our bedtime helps us phase delay, encouraging us to fall asleep and wake up later.

So for those struggling to stay awake at dinner, or anyone else who wants to fall asleep and wake up later, you actually want to get more light exposure in the four to five hours before your bedtime and avoid light first thing when you wake up.

For those who want help falling asleep and waking up earlier, the best time for daily light exposure is from the moment you wake up through the first half of your day. This can be as simple as hanging out by a window or, ideally, getting outside in the sun for at least 30 minutes first thing in the morning. Once you're at work, find ways to expose yourself to light there as well. A 2014 study shows participants with windows near their workspace "slept an average of 46 minutes more per night during the workweek than workers in workplaces without windows."

This is also crucial for the elderly, who need even more light than their younger counterparts since our eye lenses become thicker and more yellow with age, allowing less light, and especially less blue light, to reach the eye.

For anyone who doesn't have the option to get sunlight during the day, Dr. Mariana Figueiro, chief of the Rutgers Medical School Division of Sleep and Circadian Medicine, says at least 750 lux of electric light can help. A 2002 study of twelve night-shift workers showed they not only reported feeling more alert after bright light exposure during their shift, their total sleep also increased by an average of 33 minutes. Even astronauts rate bright light therapy as "highly effective."

Unfortunately those who need bright light most—like shift workers, frequent travelers, and extreme chronotypes—are also most at risk for getting it at the wrong times, because in these cases the usual instructions may not apply.

Take jet lag, for example. If you fly from the United States to Europe, it may be morning in your destination when you land, but as far as your body is concerned, it's still nighttime. So getting light in the morning would delay your clock instead of advancing it, prolonging your jet lag.

This can happen for anyone who needs to wake up at a time their body considers night or go to bed at a time their body considers morning.

The guide below, created with the help of Dr. Figuero, should help clarify when to get light and avoid light to help your sleep, no matter what your schedule. Shift workers, see chapter 14 for further guidance.

How-To: Bright Light Therapy

Warning: Bright light therapy is *not* recommended for those who have certain eye problems, bipolar disorder, or light sensitivity or those who are taking medications that cause light sensitivity, nor is it indicated for rotating shift workers who keep their schedules for less than two weeks (see the section on troubleshooting for more on that). Bright light therapy can also sometimes cause side effects like nausea, headaches, and even hypomania in rare cases. If it feels wrong, stop. As always, consult your doctor.

Preparation

- Find at least two consecutive nights (ideally more) when you can go to bed when sleepy and wake up without an alarm clock. Use this to determine your natural bedtime and natural wake time.
- Establish a realistic target bedtime and target wake time that you can stick to consistently, even on weekends.

To Shift Your Clock Earlier

1. Expose yourself to bright light, ideally sunlight, at your natural wake time for at least 30 minutes. The light must reach your eyes, but don't stare at the light source. You should not need to squint. Time this to your natural wake time regardless of when you actually wake

up. Feel free to go about any activities that don't block the light from reaching your eyes.

2. Get as much light as you can for approximately the next 8 hours.
3. Avoid unnecessary light from 5 hours before your natural bedtime until at least three hours before your natural wake time. To your body this is nighttime, so bright light now will move your clock in the wrong direction.
4. Advance your times for light exposure by up to an hour a day until you're synced up with your target schedule. If you have the option, gradually advance your wake time and sleep time as well.
5. Continue with at least 30 minutes of bright light exposure at your new wake-up time for at least another week.
6. Stick to your new wake time even on weekends. Sleeping in can cause a relapse.
7. If trying to advance 8 hours or more, consider delaying instead. Unless you're very morning oriented, it is easier to delay than advance.

To Shift Your Clock Later

1. Expose yourself to bright light in the 1 to 2 hours leading up to your natural bedtime. Time this to your natural bedtime, regardless of when you actually go to sleep. Feel free to go about any activities that don't block the light from reaching your eyes.

   • If staying up later, feel free to get extra light, provided it doesn't conflict with step 2.

2. Avoid unnecessary light from 3 hours before your natural wake time until 5 hours before your natural bedtime. To your body, this is morning, so bright light now will move your clock in the wrong direction.
3. Delay your windows for light exposure by up to an hour a day until you're synched with your target schedule. If your schedule permits, gradually delay your wake time and bedtime as well.

For Jet Lag

• If possible, start bright light therapy before your trip. This gives you a head start and reduces your risk of getting light at the wrong time upon arrival, especially when you're traveling east.

(continued on next page)

- **For Traveling East:** Follow the instructions above for shifting the clock earlier, based on your natural bedtime and wake time in your departure city.
- **For Traveling West:** Follow the instructions above for shifting the clock later, based on your natural bedtime and wake time in your departure city.

Light Timing Calculator

For a quick way to calculate your light timing for jet lag, you can also use a digital option like the Timeshifter or Entrain apps. To be clear, to my knowledge, these options have not been clinically tested, and I don't know what exact calculations they use to get their results. But Timeshifter was created by a renowned circadian rhythm researcher, Dr. Steven Lockley of Harvard Medical School, and Entrain was developed at the University of Michigan by math experts based on circadian research. Timeshifter has great reviews in the Apple App store. Your first trip is free, and then you can pay for each additional trip or for a year of unlimited trip planning. The app also includes optional advice on caffeine and melatonin timing, and it lets you plan around your flight schedule, normal sleep schedule, and chronotype. Entrain, on the other hand, uses your "lighting history, activity, and heart rate to recommend schedules of light and dark." It does not offer caffeine, melatonin, or sleep timing guidance, and it has only 2.3 stars in the Apple App store, with most negative reviews critiquing the user interface. *But* it's also free.

Shift workers should note that Timeshifter also has the Shift Work App to help users minimize the circadian effects of difficult work schedules. More on that in Chapter 14. The creator of Entrain tells me she's also working on a version for shift workers.

> **Pro Tip: Keep It Comfortable and Convenient**
>
> Many bright light boxes are 10,000 lux—aka really effing bright! This is great for some but can be uncomfortable for others and can increase the chances of side effects. Dr. Figueiro says as a general guideline, the brightness should not be so high that you're inclined to avert your eyes or squint, and as low as 750 lux at the eye can be effective.
>
> My first bright light box was the size of a large computer monitor, but the one I have now is the size of a small tablet and just sits on my desk like a picture frame. For an even more on-the-go option you can also try light therapy glasses.

THE SPECTRUM FIX:
LIGHTING COLOR/TONE

We've all heard by now that blue light before bedtime negatively impacts sleep. Then a 2019 study showed that in mice, a less studied part of the eye had a more powerful response to yellow light.

The study sparked a number of headlines positing that software that changes screens from blue to yellow in the evening is counterproductive. The researchers also suggested that contrary to popular belief, using warmer light tones in the day and cooler light tones in the evening "may be more beneficial." Their theory: Blue light is actually associated with twilight, while yellow light is associated with bright daylight.

I had a very unscientific reason to be skeptical about these suggestions. Anyone who's had to do makeup for different lighting knows that to mimic the effect of daylight, you need a white light with cold tones, not warm ones. Of course I don't expect you to take sleep tips based on my makeup mirror. So I reached out to the study's lead author, Dr. Timothy Brown, who very graciously walked me through his findings. And then I spoke to a few experts in the field, some of whose studies he actually recommended.

Based on their feedback, this research is cutting edge, but they say for now at least, the overwhelming evidence still indicates that blue light is the strongest synchronizing agent for the human circadian system. So ideally you want to be exposed to daylight or light with colder tones during the day, and then avoid blue light in the hours before bed in favor of warmer tones, or ideally no light.

Adjustable LEDs

Some lightbulbs offer multiple color options in one, where you can change from cooler tones during the day to warmer tones at night and in some cases also dim the light, with the help of an app or the flick of a switch.

Red Night-Lights

Dr. Satchin Panda, a researcher and professor at the Salk Institute for Biological Studies, also suggests using red bulbs in night-lights, which he says can be particularly helpful in a bedroom night-light that's on all night.

Still, it's important to remember that bright light of any color can prompt an alerting response. So while changing color temperature may be helpful, the much bigger emphasis should be on reducing the *amount* of light you're exposed to before bed.

THE AWARENESS FIX:
LIGHT EXPOSURE CHART

Since most of us don't walk around with a lux meter, see the chart below for a general guideline of how much light you're exposed to in different environments.

LIGHT EXPOSURE CHART		
	ENVIRONMENT	APPROXIMATE EXPOSURE
DAYTIME/ SUNLIGHT	Direct Sunlight	100,000 lux
	Daylight	10,000 lux
	Overcast	1,000 lux
	Indoors near window	1,000 lux
	Indoors away from window	25 - 50 lux
NIGHTTIME/ ELECTRIC LIGHT	Office	1,500 - 250 lux
	Operating Room	1,000 lux
	Supermarket, Workshop	750 lux
	Library, Grocery Store, Show Room, Lab	500 lux
	Kitchen	500 lux
	Gym	500 lux
	Child Care Center	500 lux
	Conference Room	300 lux
	Classroom	250 lux
	Dining Area	200 - 150 lux
	Lobby, Hallway, Stairwell, Bathroom	200 lux
	Warehouse, Home, Theater	150 lux
	Public area with dark surroundings	20 - 50 lux
	Twilight (with no electric lighting)	10 lux
	Night Sky (with no electric lighting)	0.1 lux or less
*Based on data from the National Optical Astronomy Observatory		

THE FURTHER READING FIX:
SCREEN HACKS

Unfortunately for our sleep, traditional lighting isn't our only source of evening light, and for most of us, the other one is much harder to part with: screens. But there's a lot more to consider in the discussion about screens than most sleep literature will have you believe. So see chapter 16 for more on how to best use (and not use) screens to help your sleep.

THE SHADY FIX:
SUN BLOCK

Controlling exposure to electric light in the evening is pretty simple once you have the knowledge and tools to do it. But things get a bit more difficult if your evening comes when the sun's still up, either due to shift work or because of a late sunset. Remember the study that found on average 25 lux of evening light caused a 50 percent drop in melatonin? Now consider that sunlight can hit over 100,000 lux, and you can start to understand why it can be hard to sleep shortly after being in daylight.

Luckily, there are many simple things you can do to help this problem. If you don't have to drive, wear blue-blocking or dark sunglasses while you're out and during your commute home. Ensure your bedroom is "light-tight" by following the guidance in chapter 22. And close your window coverings around the house before you leave, so your home is dark when you arrive—anything to trick your circadian rhythm into thinking it's nighttime.

This was one of the most effective things I did during my time on the overnight shift, but you don't have to take my word for it. The same twelve night workers in the study cited above reported their total sleep time increased by an average of 67 minutes after they wore dark sunglasses during their commute home—over an hour of extra sleep, just by wearing sunglasses! And that was on top of the 33 extra minutes they reported from bright light exposure. Other studies have reported similar benefits of sunglasses and blue-blocking glasses as well. And while this is especially important for anyone working an overnight shift, it can apply to anyone who doesn't feel sleepy at their desired bedtime. But again, if you have to drive home, skip the sunglasses, as they can increase your risk of falling asleep while driving.

Even now I use light management to help me function as a night owl on a morning news schedule. I close the shades and dim screens and lights in the early evening, and wear sunglasses if I'm outside before dark. These small steps help to trick my circadian rhythm into thinking it's later than it really is, so my wake-up time feels much more natural.

CHAPTER 9

The Right Way to Take Melatonin

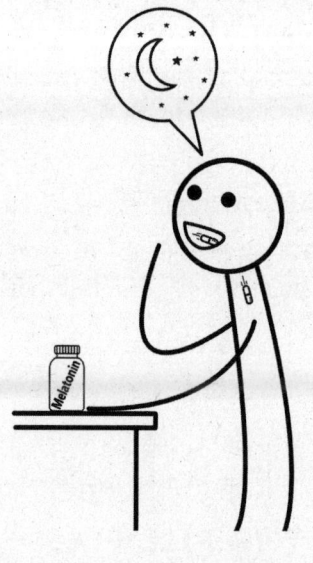

SLEEP AIDS IN GENERAL ARE misunderstood, but none more so than supplemental melatonin. Often described as a natural and non-addictive sleep aid, melatonin sounds like an insomniac's dream: pop a pill, go to sleep, fear no repercussions—problem solved. Unfortunately, the reality is a bit more complicated.

As Dr. Matthew Walker explains in his book *Why We Sleep,* melatonin is like the guy that fires the gun at the start of the race. It signals to the body that it's nighttime, but just like that guy doesn't actually run the race, melatonin doesn't generate sleep. It's like a parent telling the kids it's bedtime; unfortunately the kids might still be awake for a while. In fact, while melatonin can induce sleepiness in humans, nocturnal rodents actually become more active with melatonin. So melatonin is really a cue to engage in your typical nighttime behavior.

For most insomniacs, the issue is not that we're not getting this cue, it's that our typical nighttime behavior is staring at the ceiling feeling frustrated that we're awake. The gentle nudge of drowsiness melatonin can provide is usually not enough to get us over the hump. Hence, melatonin is not recommended as a general treatment for chronic insomnia. This can prove very frustrating for insomniacs like me who read all the hype and then find melatonin doesn't work for us. We end up thinking of ourselves as even more broken than before.

But it turns out, while melatonin isn't very effective at overpowering arousal and knocking us out, it can be very helpful when it comes to shifting our circadian rhythm. But to use it this way—you can't take it at bedtime.

THE PILL FIX:
MELATONIN FOR CIRCADIAN SHIFTING

Since light limiting and light therapy center on the body's melatonin production, you might think it would be more effective to cut out the middleman and just take melatonin. Unfortunately you would be wrong. Dr. Helen Burgess, co-director of the University of Michigan Medical School's Sleep and Circadian Research Laboratory, tells me that while well-timed bright light can shift the circadian clock by roughly an hour per day, "on average, melatonin can help shift you about half an hour a day."

Still, in certain circumstances well-timed bright light or darkness might not be an option, or you might choose to use melatonin in addition to light and dark to maximize your clock-shifting poten-tial. The guide below, created with the help of Dr. Burgess, will help clarify how to take melatonin to shift your circadian clock earlier or later.

How-To: Melatonin for Circadian Shifting

Warnings: While short-term use of melatonin is generally considered safe for most people, according to the National Institutes of Health, "there's not enough information yet about possible side effects to have a clear picture of overall safety" and "information on the long-term safety of supplementing with melatonin is lacking." There are particular concerns for diabetics, those who are pregnant and/or breastfeeding, older patients, anyone with dementia, children, and anyone taking medication, as melatonin can interact with other drugs. To help ensure you're actually getting what's on the label, look for supplements verified by ConsumerLab.com, NSF International, USP, or UL, LLC.

Preparation

- Find at least two consecutive nights (ideally more) when you can go to bed when sleepy and wake without an alarm clock. Use this to determine your natural bedtime and natural wake time.
- Establish a realistic target bedtime and target wake time that you can stick to consistently, even on weekends.

To Shift Your Clock Earlier

1. Take .5 milligram of melatonin five hours before your natural bedtime. Time this to your natural bedtime regardless of when you're actually going to bed.

Note: For most people this is not enough melatonin to induce sleepiness, but some are more sensitive. To be safe, test this out on an evening when you can safely be drowsy.

2. Shift your melatonin timing up by a half hour a day (or an hour a day if also using bright light therapy) until you're taking it five hours before your target sleep time.

(continued on next page)

- If your schedule permits, move your bedtime and wake time up by a half hour a day as well.
- If you change your sleep schedule more abruptly and your melatonin timing coincides with your new bedtime, a higher dosage of 3 to 5 milligrams may help induce sleepiness.

Note: If you are shifting more than 8 hours, consider delaying instead, as that is easier for everyone but extreme morning types.

If you can't take melatonin at your scheduled time, Burgess says within two hours "should be okay, just not optimal."

To Shift Your Clock Later

1. Take .5 mg of melatonin at your natural wake time, or within 2 hours of natural wake time if that's not an option.

    - If you wake up more than 2 hours after your natural wake time, use other options, like light, for phase delaying instead of melatonin.

2. Shift the timing of the melatonin later by a half hour a day until you reach your target wake time.

    - If your schedule permits, move your bedtime and wake time later by a half hour a day as well, until you reach your target schedule.

For Jet Lag

- If possible, start melatonin shifting before your trip. This gives you a head start and reduces your risk of getting light at the wrong time upon arrival, especially when you're traveling east.
- **For Traveling East:** Follow the instructions above for shifting the clock earlier, based on your natural bedtime and wake time in your departure city.
- **For Traveling West:** Follow the instructions above for shifting the clock later, based on your natural bedtime and wake time in your departure city.

THE PROBABLY-TOO-SUBTLE FIX:
MELATONIN FOR SLEEP ONSET

While melatonin is not recommended as a traditional sleep aid for those with insomnia, Burgess says some people may find taking it before bedtime can help them fall asleep a little bit faster. To use melatonin this way, Burgess recommends taking 3 to 5 milligrams 30 to 45 minutes before bedtime. Because the effects are subtle, she adds, "It's helpful to sort of ride the wave of melatonin" and turn in as soon as you feel drowsy. "Don't try to override it."

But since melatonin also has the power to shift circadian rhythm, it can make matters worse if used at the wrong time. So if your circadian rhythm and sleep schedule are significantly mismatched, you'll want to check the guide above to make sure you're not going to shift your clock in the wrong direction.

CHAPTER 10

Body Temperature

JUST AS MELATONIN AND CORTISOL rise and fall as part of our daily circadian rhythm, so does our core body temperature. Higher temperatures (not a fever) coincide with feeling more energized, lower temperatures (not hypothermia) coincide with feeling sleepier. So when all is in sync, our core body temperature rises around wake-up time and drops around bedtime. But if you regularly have trouble sleeping, chances are your temperature rhythms and sleep schedule are not in sync.

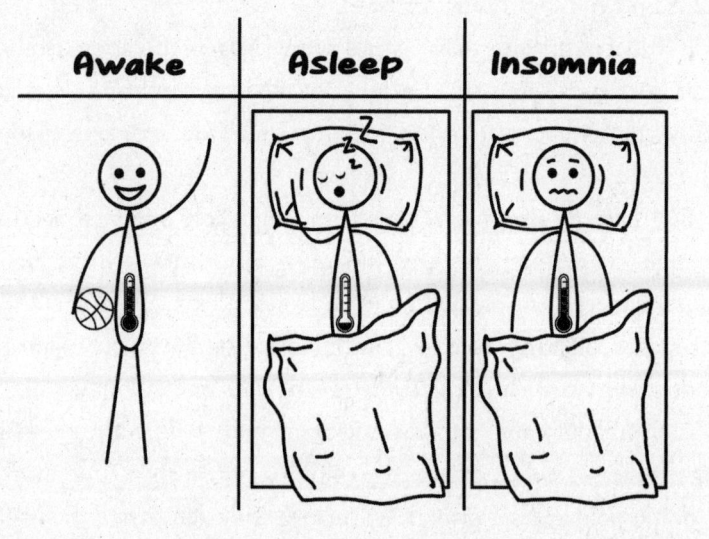

People who struggle to fall asleep tend to have a delayed temperature rhythm, so their core body temp is still too high at bedtime.

People who wake up too early tend to have an advanced temperature rhythm, so their rising body temperature wakes them up too early and keeps them awake. People who wake throughout the night tend to have elevated core body temperatures all night. And those who, like me, have trouble falling asleep and staying asleep, tend to have elevated core body temperatures *all* the time.

Sometimes this can be extreme. For example, my mother regularly wakes up feeling so hot that she gets in the shower and runs cold water on her feet to cool off. "The change in temperature in my body during the night is crazy," she tells me. "Look how desperate I get!"

Other times the changes are more subtle. My former officemate Eva Pilgrim, who co-anchors the Weekend Edition of *Good Morning America*, tells me for years she never realized how hot she was getting at night and that this was what was waking her up. It was only after I told her about my issues with body temperature that Eva started connecting the dots. "Midway through the night, I'd have kicked off the comforter," she says.

If you consistently have issues with thermoregulation, consult your doctor, as there are a number of medical conditions that can cause this. We're still trying to figure out what's causing Mom's issues.

But there are also several causes for a high core body temperature in someone perfectly healthy, including a fast metabolism, menopause, and even menstruation. Yes, ladies, along with the cramps, headaches, bloating, bleeding, and fluctuating hormones—our periods also mess with our sleep by raising core body temp (sigh).

A number of habits can also raise core body temperature, including drinking alcohol, exercising, smoking, or eating a large meal.

Some people also struggle with low body temperature, in particular low skin temperature. Dr. Roy Raymann, formerly known as Apple's "sleep czar," says this is a neglected area of the sleep temperature conversation. Raymann, now at SleepScore Labs, says low body temperature is particularly common in seniors, who tend to generate and retain less heat due to slowing metabolisms, circulatory issues, and changes in skin tissue.

Seniors also tend to have an advanced core temperature rhythm—which makes them fall asleep and wake up early. To top things off, they are less likely to notice any of these issues due to a decrease in thermosensitivity. So while you might think someone who's cold at night would just grab an extra blanket, Raymann says, "with age that doesn't happen anymore, because you just don't notice anymore."

Still, as in Eva's case, you don't have to be elderly to not realize temperature is affecting your sleep. For a long time, I too had no idea my wake-ups were due to temperature—like so many people, I thought I was waking up due to stress or to go to the bathroom (more on my temperature issues in chapter 23).

So the first step to combating body temperature issues is to look out for them. Then use the tools below to flag habits that may be contributing to them and solutions that can help get your body temperature back on track, or at least help you get better sleep despite it.

THE SURPRISING FIX:
BRIGHT LIGHT THERAPY

While the body's "master clock" largely takes its time cues from light, temperature is one of the main ways it relays those timing signals to the rest of the body. That helps to explain why temperature has such a big impact on sleep and wakefulness. It also means that if your temperature rhythm is off, there's a good chance it's due to a circadian rhythm disorder. Addressing that issue with bright light as described in chapter 8 can help not only in the long run, but according to Dr. Mariana Figueiro, bright light therapy has also been shown to have an acute effect on body temperature as well.

THE SOOTHING FIX:
WARM SHOWER/BATH

One of the fastest ways to manipulate our body temp is by taking a bath or shower. But this likely doesn't work the way that you think it does. When we feel hot or cold, what we're feeling is our skin temperature, not our core temperature—which actually have somewhat of an inverse relationship (more on this in chapter 23). Warming the skin prompts the body to send blood away from the core to the skin, which in turn cools the core. Once you get out of the shower or bath, that blood releases heat into the air, furthering that cooling effect. Cooling the skin, on the other hand, triggers a protective warming response. The body pulls blood away from the skin to the core to preserve heat. So to cool your core body temperature, you actually want to take a quick warm shower or bath before bed, not a cold one.

If you prefer to soak in the tub for a while, you'll want to give yourself a little more time to cool off afterward. That's because while you're surrounded by that hot water, blood brought to the skin's surface can't lose heat to the air. During a quick bath, this effect doesn't last long enough to affect core temp. But Raymann says if you stay in the bath for, say, 30 or 40 minutes, your core body temp will rise. For this reason, he recommends ending a long bath 1 to 2 hours before bedtime, so that your core temp has enough time to cool off.

According to a 2019 review, this technique of showering or bathing before bed is associated with improved self-rated sleep quality and sleep efficiency. The review also found that "when scheduled 1–2 hours before bedtime for as little as 10 minutes," showering or bathing was associated with "significant shortening" of the amount of time it takes to fall asleep.

THE COUNTERINTUITIVE FIX:
WARM HANDS AND FEET

Counterintuitively, warming your hands or feet (if they're cold) is another great way to help cool core body temp. Like the showering or bathing technique, this kind of tricks the body into a cooling response, sending blood away from the core to the skin and extremities. This can be as simple as running your hands under warm water, soaking your feet, or using a heating pad to warm the foot of your bed. Even just keeping an extra blanket at the foot of the bed or wearing socks to bed can help (see chapter 23 for more on that).

THE FITNESS FIX:
EXERCISE TIMING

Just as a rigorous workout will raise your heart rate, it will also raise your core body temperature—there's a reason we call it "burning calories." The problem is, unlike your heart rate, your body temperature can stay elevated for up to five hours. For most people this temperature change isn't enough to disturb sleep, but as explained in a 2019 study, "for those with insomnia, exercise too close to bedtime may have the potential to negatively impact sleep."

That said, as the Johns Hopkins University School of Medicine explains, if you give your body the right amount of time to cool off, the post-exercise drop in temperature "helps to facilitate sleepiness." But getting that timing right is tricky, because how quickly your temperature drops depends on the person and several other factors, including the intensity of the workout. The most common recommendation is to exercise at least two hours before bedtime.

Dr. Shawn Youngstedt tells me his team tested this in an as-yet-unpublished study by having normally sedentary insomniacs do moderate exercise that ended two hours before bedtime. He says for most of the subjects, the evening exercise did not impair sleep, compared to reading for an hour. But he says there were a couple of people "for whom exercise in the evening really disturbed their sleep a great deal." Again, this is despite adhering to the recommended two-hour window.

Still, Youngstedt says after you've exercised consistently for two to four weeks, a so-called training effect kicks in, which promotes sleep and also better temperature regulation. This is likely why Kofi tells me he often finishes his workout about an hour before bedtime and still has no trouble falling asleep. So ultimately Youngstedt says the best time to work out would be "whenever people are willing and able to exercise on a regular basis."

If you're more of an occasional exerciser (cough) like me (cough, cough), there are a few things to consider. For those who struggle to fall asleep, exercise done in the morning or afternoon gives your body plenty of time to cool down before bed and can have the added benefit of helping to advance your circadian clock, especially if you can get some sunlight while you're at it. (See chapter 12 for more on exercise's circadian effects.) Exercise done in the evening is trickier, but can also help with sleep onset provided you can time it so your body is cooling off near bedtime.

For those who struggle with falling asleep too early, late exercise can not only help delay your circadian clock but also raise your core temperature, helping you to immediately feel more awake until you cool off.

You can use your sleep diary to note how you sleep after working out at different times to see what works best for you.

THE EATING FIX:
NO LATE, LARGE MEAL

While you might feel lethargic after a large meal, your body is hard at work digesting all that food. That digestive process produces heat, which in turn raises your core body temperature. Thus if you eat too much food too close to bedtime, as Dr. Satchin Panda explains, it "keeps core body temperature too high for sleep."

So experiment with eating your last meal earlier or making your last meal smaller and see if that helps your sleep. This can also help with circadian rhythm and acid reflux. More on meal timing in chapters 11 and 18.

THE BEDROOM FIX:
SLEEP ENVIRONMENT

There are several things you can do to ensure your sleep environment is conducive to a sleep-friendly body temp. But, contrary to popular belief, it's not always as simple as lowering the thermostat. See chapter 23 for a full rundown of those solutions. They've even helped Mom with her body temperature issues!

THE PILL FIX:
MELATONIN

Research on how melatonin impacts body temperature is relatively limited, but it is known that one of the ways melatonin helps sleep is by inducing a dilation of the peripheral blood vessels. This draws blood and heat away from the core to the skin. According to a 2018 review, researchers believe it's this vasodilation that helps supplemental melatonin induce sleepiness, and the resulting improved sleep then helps to stabilize the temperature rhythm. The researchers especially recommend low-dose supplemental melatonin for the elderly, who often suffer from circulatory issues, and diabetics, who often suffer from a melatonin deficiency. See chapter 9 for more on melatonin, and as always, consult your doctor before taking any new supplements.

THE SOBERING FIX:
NO NIGHTCAPS

While alcohol initially causes a drop in core body temperature, that drop is later followed by a rebound spike in core body temperature. This is one of several ways alcohol helps us fall asleep, but then disturbs our sleep later in the night, and it's one of the many reasons we should avoid alcohol too close to bedtime and allow ourselves enough time to sober up before going to sleep. (More on alcohol in chapter 15.)

CHAPTER 11

Meal Timing

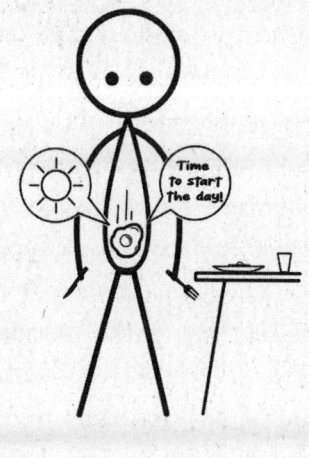

WHILE LIGHT SIGNALS THE START of the day to the brain, your first calories signal the start of the day to the gut. So for circadian rhythm, breakfast really is the most important meal of the day—but only if the meal lives up to its name: to "break" the "fast."

That's because, according to a 2019 study, the wake signal sent by our first meal of the day comes, at least in part, from a spike in the hormone insulin. But you only get that spike if you've had a long enough gap since your last meal. Like light and dark—it's all about the contrast. "So a midnight snack is a really, really bad idea," one of the researchers, Dr. John O'Neill, tells me.

That's especially interesting because sleep deprivation has been shown to increase our appetite and make us crave fat and sugar. So, stressed from being up in the middle of the night, many of us who have trouble sleeping seek comfort in a rich overnight meal. Unfortunately, not only are we setting the table for issues like indigestion, acid reflux, and weight gain—all of which negatively impact sleep—but we're also weakening our body's ability to distinguish between when we're supposed to be sleeping and when we're supposed to be awake.

And while O'Neill's studies at the UK's MRC Laboratory of Molecular Biology are primarily on mice, a few human studies on time-restricted eating or intermittent fasting show participants reported better sleep quality and duration after fasting for at least thirteen hours between their last and first meal of the day.

But there is a huge caveat to all of this that too often goes unaddressed: some of us—like me—can't fall asleep or stay asleep if we go to bed hungry. Dr. Satchin Panda, who has led several studies on time-restricted eating, tells me it's normal to have trouble sleeping due to hunger at first, but in one to three weeks, you adjust. In his book *The Circadian Code,* he writes: "You may even wake up from a deep sleep feeling hungry. Try hard to push past this by drinking a glass of water."

Still, this may be more difficult for someone who's already having sleep issues. For starters, if hunger pains can wake you from a deep sleep, imagine how much harder it is to sleep through them if you're a light sleeper. Also the common pitch from proponents of intermittent fasting is that it's not that hard to fast for twelve to sixteen hours because "you're sleeping most of that time anyway." Naturally, you lose that advantage if you're not actually sleeping most of that time.

Finally, chronic insomniacs have been shown to experience elevated cortisol levels at night, likely due to conditioned arousal or circadian rhythm issues. And guess what helps to lower cortisol? Carbs. (More on this in chapter 19.)

This isn't to say that time-restricted eating can't be helpful to people with sleep problems, but some of us may have to really ease our way in, and even Panda says, if you are using time-restricted eating to help your sleep, be sure to address issues like light, dark, noise, and habits first.

THE START HERE FIX:
PHASING OUT THE MIDNIGHT SNACK

You don't have to embrace time-restricted eating to know my meal-times were a problem. Even if my body doesn't need at least twelve hours of nighttime fasting, it's quite clear it was not designed to eat and sleep at the same time. Thus stuffing my face during my equiv-alent of the "middle of the night" definitely wasn't relaying to my circadian rhythm that this was supposed to be sleep time.

But when I was suffering from the worst of my insomnia, eating was one of the few things that brought me comfort. So I decided this was not a good area for me to rip off the proverbial Band-Aid. For once, I was going to embrace the old "slow and steady" approach.

My main problem was that during my normal day I eat every three to four hours. But due to trouble falling asleep or staying asleep, I often found myself awake three to four hours after my last meal. Just like during the day, I was hungry. And trying to sleep through these hunger pains was impossible. Maybe I would have adjusted if I'd stuck it out, as Panda suggests. But even if I'd known that at the time, I'm not sure I would have been willing to take on yet another sleep obstacle. So I took a different approach: I focused on food quality and quantity as a starting point.

Usually, when searching for a "midnight snack" I just tried to find the fastest thing I could put in my face that would taste good and make me feel good. That rarely resulted in eating something healthy. So I set out to find something satisfying, quick to prepare, and easy to have on hand that wouldn't trigger my acid reflux. My answer ended up being either a piece of whole grain toast with a little butter or plain oatmeal with a dash of salt and cinnamon, and a little honey or applesauce for sweetening. These are still my go-tos on the rare occasion I wake up at night feeling hungry, and I now know the complex carbs are also conducive to helping me fall back asleep (more on that in chapter 19).

Gradually, as my sleep improved, these middle-of-the-night awakenings happened less and less. As they did, I started paying closer attention and asking myself, *Am I actually hungry, or do I just want some comfort because I can't sleep?* If after having some water I still feel genuine hunger, I eat my snack. If not, I skip it and instead read or do something else relaxing until I feel sleepy again.

THE OFFICIAL FIX:
TIME-RESTRICTED EATING

Time-restricted eating (TRE) is pretty straightforward, but it's not always easy. To help ensure success, Panda suggests a gradual approach. Below are some instructions from his book *The Circadian Code* summarized with his approval.

How-To: Time-Restricted Eating

1. Establish a 12-hour calorie window and consume your first and last calorie of the day within those hours. Earlier in the day is preferable, and it's best to have your last meal at least 2 hours before bed, but "any schedule you can follow is better than no schedule at all."
2. For the first two weeks, eat whenever you want within your eating window, but after that, try to stick to regularly scheduled meals, especially for your first and last meals of the day.
3. After 1 to 3 weeks, try to decrease your eating window by an hour a week until you reach your goal. Panda tells me 8 hours is ideal, but he recommends 10 hours for a more feasible long-term target. He says you can also do 8 hours as an "intervention" for a few weeks and then go back to a 10-, 11-, or 12-hour window for the long term.
4. What you can have outside your window:

   • Water is always allowed, as it has no calories. It can also help you feel less hungry.

- Herbal tea before bed is also fine, but only if it has no caffeine and nothing added to it like sweetener or milk.
- Medications should be taken per your doctor's orders, but some work better when taken at specific times of day. Talk to your doctor to ensure you're taking your meds at the best times.

5. Alcohol counts as calories. No booze outside of your window.
6. Coffee counts! Do not drink it outside your calorie window. If you absolutely can't resist, have it black—no milk or sweetener.
7. If you get off track, don't panic. Just get back on track as soon as you can.
8. Chart your progress (perhaps in your sleep diary). Maybe a 12-hour window is giving you the results you want. Maybe you find a tighter window to be more effective. *Note:* It's normal to plateau at times and then suddenly start seeing progress again. Don't get discouraged.

I will also add that, based on my own experience, if twelve hours doesn't seem feasible, start with a target that does and go from there. Even now, sometimes I stay within twelve hours; sometimes it's closer to thirteen. I find that works just fine for me. Do what works for you.

THE ANECDOTAL FIX: FASTING FOR JET LAG/SHIFT WORK

While time-restricted eating is all about establishing a routine, its most interesting potential benefit comes when routine isn't possible—for example, due to jet lag or rotating shift work.

When food is readily available, light and darkness run the show in setting circadian rhythm. But according to a 2008 study, "if animals have access to food only during their normal sleep cycle, they will shift most of their circadian rhythms to match the food availability." Translation: If mice fast long enough, their first meal of the day effectively resets their circadian rhythm.

For Jet Lag

The lead researcher on that study, Dr. Clifford Saper, theorizes that this could be a potential tool to combat jet lag. The thinking is, if you fast for twelve to sixteen hours, then start eating again at breakfast time in your new time zone, your circadian rhythm will adjust accordingly. Especially if you combine that with appropriately timed exposure to light and darkness.

Saper, chair of neurology at Beth Israel Deaconess Medical Center and a professor at Harvard Medical School, tells me the fasting theory needs to be clinically studied on humans to confirm it works. He adds it's possible those who try in-flight fasting simply feel better because, in lieu of eating, they're getting more sleep on the plane.

Still, many frequent travelers now swear by fasting as the ultimate weapon against jet lag. And barring any issues like an eating disorder, Saper tells me, "I don't think there's any harm in trying it."

For Shift Work

Dr. John O'Neill, whose research on insulin I previously mentioned, says his and Saper's findings could have even bigger implications for shift workers who rotate shifts or adjust their schedules on the weekends. As he puts it, "I would anticipate when you're going on to the night shift that what you should do is food-deprive yourself for at least twelve, ideally even sixteen hours, before breakfast tonight." He also advises avoiding bright light all day, and then seeing bright light as you eat breakfast around the start of your shift. "It's basically just sending signals at the right time to help your natural biological rhythm," he adds.

Just remember to stay hydrated, as dehydration can make jet lag or shift work disorder worse. As Saper explains, water doesn't reset the clock, calories do—so drink up.

THE TESTED FIX:
THE ARGONNE DIET/JET LAG PROGRAM

If you want something with more human evidence, check out the Argonne diet, created at the U.S. Department of Energy's Argonne National Laboratory back in the 1980s. The system of strategically timed sleep, meals, and caffeine was tested in 2002 on nearly 200 National Guard troops. Compared to the rest of the group, those who followed the diet were 7.5 times less likely to have jet lag on deployment and over 16 times less likely to experience jet lag returning home.

The diet is now rumored to be used by everyone from the military to the CIA. And while it's technically aimed at reducing jet lag, it also has been reported to help shift workers.

How-To: Argonne Diet

The Argonne diet is more like a program than a diet. In fact, its creator, Dr. Charles Ehret, called it "The Three-Step Jet Lag Program." Below is a short summary of the program, but you can find more detailed instructions in Ehret's book, cowritten with Lynne Waller Scanlon, called *Overcoming Jet Lag*, later retitled *The Cure for Jet Lag*.

1. Determine how many times zones you're crossing. That many days before your departure, stop consuming caffeine outside the hours of 3:00 to 4:30 P.M.
2. One to three days before the flight (depending on how many time zones you're crossing), start alternating feast days and fast days. Feast days include a high-protein breakfast, a high-protein lunch, and a high-carbohydrate dinner. Fast days include small light meals totaling roughly 800 calories for the day. If you are traveling five or more time zones, time this so you're fasting on flight day. Otherwise time this so you're feasting on flight day.

(continued on next page)

One Day Before Your Flight

- **Caffeine:** If traveling west or more than ten time zones, no caffeine outside the hours of 7:00 to 11:00 A.M. If traveling east up to two time zones, have caffeine right after 6:00 P.M. Otherwise, no caffeine outside 3:00 to 4:30 P.M.
- **Meals:** If traveling more than five time zones east, no post-dinner snacks. More than five time zones west, light snack after dinner allowed.
- **Bedtime:** If shifting eastbound more than eight time zones, try to go to bed earlier than usual.

On Departure Day

- **Sleep Schedule:** If traveling east, wake up earlier than usual. If traveling west five or more time zones, sleep as late as possible.
- **Meals:** If traveling up to four time zones, eat on destination time. Five time zones or more, stop eating a few hours before breakfast in your destination, then break your fast by eating a high-protein breakfast on your destination time.
- **Drinking:** No alcohol on the plane, but drink plenty of water.
- **Caffeine:** If you're traveling west, have caffeine in the morning. If you're traveling east up to four time zones, have no caffeine; five to ten time zones, have caffeine at 6:00 P.M. in your departure city. If you are traveling eleven to twelve time zones in either direction, have caffeine in the morning and between 7:00 and 11:30 A.M. in your departure city.

3. On arrival, try to eat, sleep, and be active in accordance with the time in your destination.

CHAPTER 12

When to Work Out

RIGHT NOW, AS YOU READ this book, even if you're just sitting on the couch, your muscles are at work. Without us even thinking about it our heart beats, our digestive tract moves food through our body, and our lungs keep us breathing. And as Dr. Satchin Panda explains, all three of those functions have a rhythm, increasing during the day and slowing at night so the body can cool down and prepare for sleep.

But just as eating can either aid or disrupt that rhythm, exercise can too.

THE EARLY FIX:
EXERCISE TO ADVANCE CIRCADIAN RHYTHM

A 2019 study examined the effect of exercise on over a hundred adults between eighteen and seventy-five years old. It found that exercise at 7:00 A.M. helped to advance their melatonin onset by almost an hour. But even more surprisingly, so did exercise between 1:00 and 4:00 P.M., with the effect diminishing only slightly in the late afternoon. That follows a 2003 study, which also found evidence that early evening exercise could advance circadian rhythm.

Dr. Shawn Youngstedt, who led the more recent study, tells me this is especially good news for struggling night owls, who would benefit from advancing their circadian rhythm, but might not be willing or able to exercise in the morning. Instead, he says, they can try exercising in the afternoon to help advance their body clock. He adds this could also help with jet lag for someone traveling east, or even social jet lag, as exercise on a Sunday afternoon could help get you back on your weekday schedule.

As for how to translate this for extreme chronotypes or odd schedules, Youngstedt says he expects that exercise within the first one to two hours after awakening and seven to ten hours before bedtime will advance the clock.

THE LATE FIX:
EXERCISE TO DELAY CIRCADIAN RHYTHM

If you are looking to delay your clock instead, Youngstedt's study suggests your best bet is to work out between 7:00 P.M. and 10:00 P.M., which delayed melatonin onset by roughly forty to fifty minutes. For those with odd hours, aim for up to four hours before bedtime.

Youngstedt says this could prove helpful for those traveling west and for anyone else looking to fall asleep and wake up later.

Overnight exercise can also prove helpful for shift workers. A 1995 study showed shift workers who cycled for fifteen minutes every hour during the first three of eight consecutive night shifts were more likely to have a large delay in temperature rhythm, compared to the control group. What's more, early birds in the control group had more difficulty delaying than night owls, as expected. But surprisingly in the exercise group, early birds were able to shift just as easily as the night owl chronotypes.

Youngstedt's study also showed exercise at 1:00 A.M. and 4:00 A.M. correlated with delays, but they were milder compared to delays from the 7:00 to 10:00 P.M. exercise. He says for night shift workers, a good general guideline to help delay circadian rhythm is to exercise during the couple of hours before or after your shift starts.

But taking into account the overall benefits of exercise, sleep experts and health experts in general seem to agree: the best time to exercise is still the time you're most likely to do it. (See chapter 10 for more on how exercise affects our body temperature.)

CHAPTER 13

Sleep Debt Strategies

GIVEN THE ADVICE IN CHAPTER 7 about consistent wake times, and the advice in chapter 5 against sleeping in, napping, or going to bed early, you might be thinking: *What about sleep debt?* This is one of the most hotly debated topics in sleep.

On the one hand, there's the "you can *never* catch up on sleep" crowd, who make it sound like you're doomed after even one night of insufficient sleep. I'm happy to report that the data doesn't support this. A landmark study from the University of Chicago, for example, restricted volunteers to only four hours of sleep for six days in a row. Over the course of the week, their blood pressure and stress hormone levels rose, they produced fewer antibodies when given a flu vaccine, and they showed signs of insulin resistance—a precursor to diabetes. But once they were allowed to recover that lost sleep, all of those changes reversed. Other studies have also shown this ability to quickly recover from suspected sleep debt-related ailments.

And while we can't ethically test the impact of longer-term sleep deprivation on humans, four hours of sleep is far less than most insomniacs get on a bad night, let alone for six days in a row. The ability to reverse the impact of that in less than a week is no small feat. As someone who has recovered from a long stint of sleep deprivation, I can tell you I was pleasantly surprised at how quickly my body bounced back. And I'm not alone.

ABC News producer Kevin Freeman tells me after four years of struggling to sleep on the overnight shift, he had so much joint pain he was tested for arthritis, was so lethargic he was tested for Lyme disease, and feared he might have a serious dental problem. "I was consistently in pain, with food lodging in my gums," he tells me. His dentist attributed the problem to age, and Kevin figured age probably explained everything else he was feeling too.

But after switching to a new show with a daytime schedule, Kevin says he's now sure all his symptoms were actually due to years of sleep deprivation. More importantly, they're now gone. "After a few months, all of these symptoms went away," he says.

I had a similar experience with my acid reflux and dry eyes. These issues that for years I accepted as a permanent part of my life, vanished surprisingly quickly once I started sleeping better.

And again, there's Jason Karp's story from chapter 2. For eight weeks he purposely limited himself to two to four hours of sleep a day. He experienced a host of extreme symptoms from skin conditions to hair loss; he even started losing his vision. But once Jason started sleeping and eating better, his symptoms started disappearing—including his supposedly incurable eye condition.

All that said, some people talk about repaying "sleep debt" as if we have some sleep account we can withdraw from, then make deposits whenever we want to break even. I'm sorry to report that this is also not true.

When it comes to paying it back, sleep debt is more like diet. If you missed a meal every day for a week, you wouldn't then eat seven extra meals in a day to make up your calorie deficit. If you did, not only would you feel terrible, but you'd likely be incapable of eating that much in one shot. And trying to force down that much food would likely ruin your appetite for a while, leading you to skip meals—perpetuating the original problem.

The same can happen with sleep. For example, let's say you

needed eight hours of sleep per day, and only got six hours a day for a week. Dr. Michael Grandner, director of the Sleep and Health Research Program at the University of Arizona College of Medicine, tells me, "You don't now need to sleep fourteen hours [all at once] to get back to baseline. If anything, if you did that, you'd feel bad." You'd also throw off your circadian rhythm. And if you spend a lot of time awake in bed trying to force those fourteen hours of sleep, you'll likely give yourself insomnia.

Instead follow the tools below for strategies on recovering a sleep debt without messing with your circadian rhythm or your sleep drive.

THE NOT-SO-FAST FIX:
FIX SLEEP DISORDERS FIRST

Trying to recover a long-term sleep debt while suffering from a sleep disorder is like trying to do physical therapy on a broken arm. First you have to fix the break. *Then* you can work on regaining your strength. In the same way, first you have to address the root causes of your sleep problems. For example, insomniacs should go back to part 2 of this book and address their arousal and sleep drive issues. Only once that's resolved should you even think about strategies for extra recovery sleep.

THE MORNING FIX:
45-MINUTE SLEEP-IN

While it's generally advised to wake up at the same time every day, in his book *The Power of When*, Dr. Michael Breus says if you sleep in for less than an hour on weekends, you're "statistically safe" from circadian-related negative effects. So if you have a rough night or rough week, set the alarm for, at most, 45 minutes after your usual wake time to avoid confusing your circadian rhythm.

THE NIGHTTIME FIX:
EARLIER BEDTIME

If an extra 45 minutes isn't going to cut it or you're the type of person who can't sleep in, the National Sleep Foundation recommends going to bed earlier instead. This is less likely to interfere with your ability to sleep the next day. But don't go overboard. The foundation suggests "backing up your bedtime by 15 minutes per night to gradually shift your body's clock." More importantly, don't go to bed earlier if you don't feel sleepy.

If the early bedtime interferes with your ability to fall asleep or stay asleep, adhere to stimulus control rules explained in chapter 5 and resume your normal sleep schedule going forward.

THE MIDDAY FIX:
NAPPING

Napping is another alternative to reducing sleep debt, but timing matters here too. Dr. Helen Burgess recommends waking up at your usual time and staying up for at least two hours, as this is when we "get the most bang for our buck" from light exposure. She says after that you can take a nap without much impact to your circadian rhythm because you've already given your clock that morning light to sync to.

That said, napping too long or too late can still interfere with our sleep drive, making it hard to sleep at bedtime. The National Sleep Foundation recommends going for a 20-minute power nap, or if you're looking for a longer snooze, aiming for 60 to 90 minutes.

If you find the nap does interfere with your sleep, adhere to stimulus control rules explained in chapter 5 and try shortening the nap next time or skipping it altogether.

THE BEHIND THE SCENES FIX:
AUTO SLEEP RECOVERY

While it's annoying that you can't just withdraw and deposit sleep like money, there's a big silver lining to that: you also don't have to pay it all back. When we're sleep deprived, our body automatically prioritizes deep sleep and REM sleep over lighter, less restorative stages of sleep. We also fall asleep faster than usual and sleep more efficiently.

So after a period of sleep deprivation, even if you go back to spending only your usual amount of time in bed, you still get more deep sleep, more REM sleep, and more overall sleep than you usually would. In other words, as long as we don't get in the way, over time our body will pay back sleep debt automatically.

This should come as a relief to anyone who, like me, has a hard time going to bed early or napping, even when sleep-deprived. If attempts at extra recovery sleep aren't working, don't force it. It's probably a sign your body is already doing the work for you.

It's also worth noting, as explained in chapter 4, that insomniacs tend to underestimate how much sleep they get. So if your problem is insomnia, chances are your sleep debt isn't as bad as you think it is.

CHAPTER 14

The Graveyard Shift

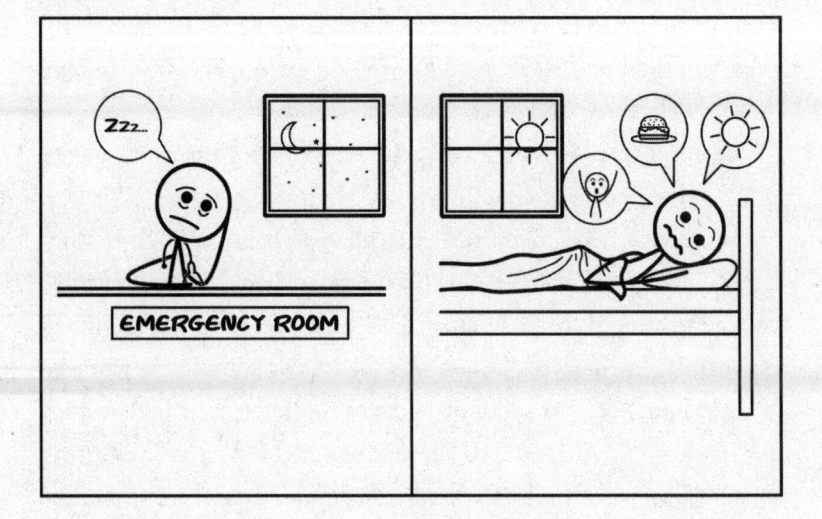

WHEN IT COMES TO CIRCADIAN rhythm issues, one group of people are in a league of their own: those who work overnight hours, aka the graveyard shift. Graveyard shift workers are particularly vulnerable to sleep and health issues because our work schedules conflict so drastically with our circadian rhythm. We get home and go to bed, but our circadian rhythm is telling our body it's time to be awake. So of course we have trouble sleeping. Then when we get to work, we're not only sleep-deprived, but our circadian rhythm is also telling our body it's bedtime—a double whammy of sleepiness that can sometimes last the whole shift. To get through this, we chug coffee, especially toward the end of the shift as we start to get sleepier. Come morning when our shift ends, our circadian wake drive rises again. That plus the caffeine makes it hard to sleep. Rinse and repeat. Welcome to shift work disorder.

There are plenty of articles and books describing the scenario above and explaining why it's so bad for you. But there's very little out there presenting solutions other than: quit your job. Part of the reason for that may be that very few medical studies focus on shift work—ironic given the fact that a huge component of the shift working community is medical workers! If you needed emergency surgery in the middle of the night, wouldn't you want your surgeon to be as well rested and alert as possible?

The good news is there's still a lot we can do with what science has already uncovered about circadian rhythms.

But we also need to address the other problem with shift work that often goes untold: the unspoken expectation that we somehow manage to sleep during the daytime—and also fulfill a long list of responsibilities then too. When was the last time someone working daytime hours had to wake up in the middle of the night to pick up the kids, take their pet to the vet, or see the dentist? You think it's annoying when the repairman tells you he'll be there sometime between 11:00 A.M. and 3:00 P.M.? Imagine if he told you he'd be there between 11:00 P.M. and 3:00 A.M.! That's what it's like to be a shift worker. ALL. THE. TIME.

The rest of our world is awake and bustling. That means our sleep is often disturbed by light and noise, but also by social obligations, work obligations, even just the simple knowledge that there are a million things we could be doing other than sleeping.

And despite the overwhelming health issues we always hear so much about, for shift workers, even seeing the doctor becomes a challenge. Call to get an appointment and you hear the equivalent of "She can see you at 1:00 A.M. or 4:00 A.M." Not the best scenario for someone whose main issue is lack of sleep.

So yes, biology makes it hard to sleep when you're trying to be nocturnal, but so does the fact that daytime sleep just isn't respected or protected the same way nighttime sleep is. The Fixes below aim to help with both problems.

THE MINDSET FIX:
SLEEP TIME, NOT FREE TIME

This may sound stupid, but the first step to sleeping during the day is *choosing* to sleep. For people who sleep at night, this choice is fairly automatic, because everyone else is sleeping too.

For those who sleep during the day, however, this becomes a conscious decision, because there are so many alternative options. We're also so used to the idea that daytime is for productivity, that sleeping during the day feels selfish or lazy. This is perhaps best illustrated by the number of times shift workers are asked, "What do you do with all your free time during the day?" Note to day workers: We hate that question. But we also often espouse the same idea—that our daytime hours are free time. Step one is to make the active decision that an adequate window of your day is not free time, it's sleep time, and that's no more negotiable than everyone else's sleep time at night.

THE CUSTOM FIX:
CONSIDER YOUR CHRONOTYPE

Just as different chronotypes are naturally inclined to different bedtimes at night, the same is true during the day. So if you haven't already, see chapter 6 to figure out your chronotype. For night owls, circadian rhythm is still low in the early morning hours. So shift work sleep consultant Carolyn Schur recommends that this group go home after their night shift and try to sleep as soon as possible. Early bird types, on the other hand, can find it very difficult to sleep in the morning, because that's when their circadian rhythm is naturally higher. Instead, Schur recommends that these people go to sleep later in the day, or at least wait until later in the morning, "maybe nine-thirty or ten."

This worked well for me when I was exclusively on *World News Now* and *America This Morning*. My shift was always over by 6:00 A.M., so as a night owl, I just viewed it as a really late night. I'd get home, go straight to bed, and get a consistent 6 to 7 hours.

My former producer, Janine Elliot, on the other hand, describes herself as more of a morning person. Unsurprisingly, Janine has better luck sleeping from 11:30 A.M. to 7:30 P.M.

THE STEADY FIX:
CONSISTENCY

Once I started having trouble sleeping during the day, I became very jealous of Janine's unwavering 8+ hours. I always thought it was just biology, that she was just a "good sleeper." But while biology can certainly help, in all my interviews with various night shift workers, those who sleep best all share something in common: a consistent routine.

I botched this big-time.

After I started making regular appearances on *Good Morning America*, my strategy was still to sleep as soon as I got home. But that meant going to bed around 6:00 A.M. on days I didn't have *GMA*, and as late as 10:00 A.M. on days I did (my eating schedule was just as erratic). The late days were really tough and I slept really badly, so the early morning days felt like a good opportunity to catch up on that lost sleep. But soon, even on 6:00 A.M. days, I'd lie in bed, tired, frustrated, and awake. It was only when I chose consistency and started staying up until at least 9:00 A.M. regardless of my work schedule, and getting up by 5:00 P.M. regardless of how much I slept, that my sleep finally started to improve (see chapter 5 for more on this). This was possibly the worst time to sleep for my circadian rhythm, but I knew that sleeping later in the day would mean never seeing my husband or friends. As a very social person, I knew that would have psychological repercussions and decided it wasn't worth the trade-off.

The good news is, my body adjusted to the schedule anyway—thanks to consistency and some of the other Fixes detailed throughout this book. It's another reminder that all of these tools are meant to be used in the way that makes the most sense for you.

I've found it also helps to think of your sleep and wake times as if they were still night and morning, and then conduct your day accordingly. For example, Janine says during the week she thinks of her 11:30 A.M. bedtime as 11:30 P.M., and her 7:30 P.M. wake time as 7:30 A.M. "I have breakfast, go to the gym . . . I bring lunch to work and eat dinner when I go home . . . just like I would if I worked normal hours," she tells me. Andrea Grymes, my old co-anchor at CBS New York, did the same. "It helped to treat my 1:30 A.M. wake-up time like it was 6:30 A.M. and eat dinner when I got home" around 2:00 P.M., she tells me. It makes sense now why Andrea functioned so much better on that shift than I did.

Still, for some, this consistency might have to entail two blocks of sleep, rather than one. If this is the case, try to make one block at least six hours. The more sequential sleep you can get, the better.

ABC overnight producer Jack Sheahan tells me despite getting off work at 5:00 A.M., he doesn't go to sleep until 11:00 A.M. on weekdays. He then wakes up around 5:00 P.M., has dinner, watches the news, and then goes *back* to bed from 7:00 to 8:30 P.M. Jack says this process has served him well for twenty-five years of overnight work. But he says the key to his success is consistency, adding, "If things get thrown off . . . it could be a rough couple days until routine can be established again."

THE ACCELERATED FIX:
CIRCADIAN SHIFTING

Consistency alone will help your circadian rhythm adjust to your new schedule, but using tools like well-timed exercise (see chapter 12), meals (see chapter 11), melatonin (see chapter 9), and most of all, light exposure (see chapter 8) will help to not only ensure that happens but also make it happen more quickly. So be sure to read all of part 3 of this book to get a good idea of all the circadian shifting tools at your disposal. If you intend to try to keep more "normal" hours on the weekends, see the next Fix to help you pick the best circadian position for you.

For a quick way to get custom guidance on circadian shifting, you can also check out the Shift Work App by Timeshifter. According to the company, the app uses your schedule, sleep pattern, chronotype, and preferences to provide personalized recommendations for when to do things like get or avoid light, consume caffeine, and/or take melatonin to minimize circadian disruptions. As of the writing of this book, the app is set to launch October 2021, and an annual subscription will cost $149. It will also be available for a monthly subscription, and both options will include a two-week free trial.

THE REALISTIC FIX:
WHAT TO DO ABOUT WEEKENDS

It's one thing to be up all night with your coworkers and then sleep while your family is at work or school. It's a whole new challenge to be up all night by yourself tiptoeing around the house, and then sleep all day when your family is either home or out having fun. Trust me, I know from experience.

This is why most shift workers try to keep more normal hours on weekends, but this can result in *severe* social jet lag. So how do you shift off the zombie hours without screwing everything up?

Build Up Sleep Drive

The most straightforward way to successfully shift your sleep schedule is to build up your sleep drive at the right times. Jack does this by sleeping only two hours on Friday afternoon, so he's accumulated enough sleep pressure to sleep again from roughly 10:00 P.M. to 6:00 A.M. Then on Saturdays he tries to stay up late and wake again at 6:00 A.M. Come Sunday afternoon, he sleeps from 1:30 to 5:30 P.M. and again from 7:00 to 8:30 P.M. Jack tells me, "By this point I believe my body knows that by Sunday afternoon, I'll be lying down again to rest, and it's almost an autopilot thing."

ABC correspondent Trevor Ault says he used to build up his sleep drive before his Friday split shift at WTOL in Toledo, Ohio, where he had to work from 4:00 A.M. to 8:00 A.M., and then again from 5:00 P.M. until roughly midnight. "At first I would just power through and just try to stay awake, but you realize that when that 11:30 live shot comes around, you look like a zombie, even if you think your brain is functioning," Trevor said.

To troubleshoot this, Trevor knew he needed to take a nap in the middle of the day, but coming off his normal schedule, he wasn't able to fall asleep. So he eventually figured out that if he stayed up later than usual on Thursday night and woke up earlier than usual on Friday morning, his sleep drive would be high enough come late Friday morning that he could get a nap in before going back in at five. "That's the only way you get it to work," he says.

Janine also swears by building up sleep drive, but she does it through exercise. "On Sundays I always work out in the morning so that I'm tired enough to sleep for at least four or so hours in the afternoon leading up to my shift," she tells me, "That helps me adjust back to the overnight schedule."

Compromise Circadian Position

During my time on the overnight shift, keeping a different sleep schedule on weekends did not work well for me. Switching from daytime to nighttime sleep was a breeze. It was like my body recognized this familiar place and settled right in. Switching back on Sundays was a whole other story, mainly because I'm a terrible napper. My sleep drive has to be very high for me to sleep during the day. Without a nap on Sunday, I was beyond exhausted at work. So I'd load up on caffeine to get through the night. That plus my high circadian wake drive would screw up my sleep when I got home in the morning and kick off a bad cycle.

I wish I'd known then about what researchers call a compromise circadian phase position. This is what happens when you shift your circadian rhythm halfway between your weekday schedule and weekend schedule. According to a series of studies that culminated in 2009, subjects who were partially entrained this way showed "markedly improved mood, fatigue, and performance" during night shifts compared to control groups. Add to that, those who were partially entrained actually showed comparable impairment levels to those whose circadian rhythms were fully entrained to the night shift. A 2008 study also found that even when their compromise circadian positions were slightly off the target, partially entrained subjects "were able to sleep for almost all of the scheduled time both after night shifts and on days off."

Exactly how to achieve a compromise circadian phase position will depend on factors like your schedule and chronotype. But here's a general guide I created with the help of Dr. Helen Burgess.

How-To: Compromise Circadian Position

1. Determine your weekday and weekend sleep schedules, aiming to maintain at least three overlapping hours (but preferably more). For example, someone who sleeps from 7:00 A.M. to 3:00 P.M. during the week might make their weekend sleep schedule 3:00 A.M. to 11:00 A.M.
2. Find the midpoint between your weekday and weekend bedtimes. This is your circadian bedtime. Do the same for your wake times.
3. Follow the guidelines for bright light therapy from chapter 8, and/or melatonin timing from chapter 9, using your circadian bedtime and wake time as your "targets."
4. If you have trouble waking up on your days off, 30 minutes of bright light upon waking will help you shift a little earlier and feel more alert.
5. If possible, napping before your shift can be helpful, especially before your first night back.
6. If needed, consider having caffeine in the first 2 hours of your night shift to improve alertness, especially on your first night back.

Of course, circadian shifting takes time, so Burgess says this works best if you're working the night shift for at least two weeks. Those whose work schedules change rapidly won't be able to shift in time. But researchers have also suggested that a compromise circadian position might be helpful for rotating shift workers whose schedules change slowly.

When done properly, this significantly reduces your social jet lag, making it that much easier to adjust to your weekend schedule, and more importantly, to readjust when it's time to go back to the overnight shift.

THE COMPLICATED FIX:
CAFFEINE

As you'll learn in chapter 17, caffeine is a complicated beast, but even more so for shift workers. On the one hand, caffeine has been shown to reduce errors and improve cognitive performance in shift workers. On the other hand, it's also been shown to have a stronger negative effect on daytime sleep compared to nighttime sleep. Based on various studies, it seems the best way to balance this is to limit caffeine use to within the first two to three hours of a night shift.

As for dosage, it obviously varies based on each person's sensitivity, but research has shown 1.8 milligrams of caffeine per pound of body weight decreased sleepiness on the overnight shift for 6 hours in one study and 7.5 hours in another, and was effective in both mild and moderate caffeine users. For reference, an average cup of coffee has roughly 100 milligams of caffeine.

That said, caffeine is not an adequate replacement for sufficient sleep. Not only do we develop a tolerance to caffeine when we use it daily, but a 2017 study found when subjects were restricted to only five hours of sleep a night, the benefits of caffeine wore off after just three nights.

So consider using caffeine more as a short-term performance enhancer to get you back on track, rather than using it as a daily necessity.

THE DOUBLE-EDGED FIX:
NAPPING

Napping is often touted as one of the best ways to deal with night work, and for good reason. It has been shown to not only decrease sleepiness and boost alertness on a night shift, but also help "prevent adverse effects due to night shift work"—including car accidents. This is especially helpful when circadian entrainment isn't possible, like in rapidly rotating shift work, or ahead of your first night shift after some time off.

But what often goes unmentioned is, according to a 2005 study, "the length of daytime sleep after [a] night shift, when combined with a nighttime nap, is shorter than that without [a] nap." You will have to decide whether you consider that a pro or a con.

Also, as I mentioned, some of us nap more easily than others. For myself, I've learned to see naps as a period of rest, where sleep is a bonus, not an expectation, because sleep doesn't usually happen for me in this context. So banking on being able to get extra sleep in the form of a nap may not work for everyone.

For the many people who do rely on napping, keep in mind that we fall into deep sleep more quickly if napping while sleep-deprived. This helps reduce sleep debt, but waking up out of deep sleep can leave you with really bad sleep inertia. That means you'll be groggy and impaired until your brain can fully wake up again. Researchers believe circadian rhythm also affects sleep inertia, another reason we may be more susceptible to sleep inertia when napping overnight. Finally, the length of a nap is crucial. A 2014 study found a 30-minute nap during a night shift produced sleep inertia that lasted up to 45 minutes, but a 10-minute nap helped workers' performance with little to no sleep inertia. And these participants were well rested, and thus less likely to experience sleep inertia compared to most night shift workers.

So if you're taking a nap before a night shift, Dr. Chris Winter, a neurologist and sleep specialist, says do your best to stick to a schedule, give yourself at least a half hour before you get in the car, and expose yourself to light, heat, physical activity, and social interaction upon waking.

If you're taking a nap during a night shift, keep it short, and take it at the beginning of your break to leave as much time as possible to recover from potential sleep inertia before going back to work.

You might also consider having a quick dose of caffeine before the nap to help further minimize potential sleep inertia. (See chapter 17 for more on that.)

THE DEFENSIVE FIX:
PROTECT YOUR SLEEP

No matter how primed your body is for daytime sleep, you won't be successful if that sleep is constantly interrupted by light, noise, or any other outside factors. Ensuring your bedroom is completely dark and otherwise conducive to sleep is a good place to start and is especially important for daytime sleepers. (See part 5 for more on that.)

But daytime sleepers will also have additional interruptions that nighttime sleepers don't have to think about. For me, this was phone calls. People don't call you overnight unless it's an emergency, but you never notice how much your phone rings during the day until it happens while you're trying to sleep. I was constantly woken up by everything from appointment confirmations to robocalls about my car insurance—even though I don't own a car. Once I was even woken up by my doctor's office, ironically telling me I was otherwise healthy and just needed to get more sleep. Thanks!

The most common advice I heard was to silence my phone. But I needed to be reachable for work, and I didn't like the idea of not being reachable to family and friends in case of emergency. Eventually, I discovered the "Do Not Disturb" phone setting, which allows for only certain calls to ring. I still have my phone set to automatically go on "Do Not Disturb" from my bedtime until my wake time. That means my family or my office can still get through to me, but I don't get calls about the warranty for the car I still don't own.

The American Academy of Sleep Medicine also suggests putting up an actual DO NOT DISTURB sign on your door, temporarily disconnecting your doorbell, and making sure your household knows you're sleeping.

Pro Tip: Don't Forget the Doorman

Apartment dwellers, notify your doorman or super of your sleep schedule as well so they know not to disturb you.

Finally, I also sought to eliminate sleep-disturbing appointments by finding professionals who could work around my sleep schedule, like doctors who had early or late hours and were comfortable communicating over email-like platforms instead of making me call during regular business hours. This meant I could not only see the doctor without disrupting my sleep schedule but also request an appointment or ask a quick question without disrupting my sleep schedule. And while telemedicine is now widely accepted thanks to the Covid-19 pandemic, it was a novelty when my sleep doctor offered it to me, and a much-appreciated one. It saved me the time of commuting to his office, and allowed him to take late appointments from home—which meant I didn't have to skip sleep to see the sleep doctor.

Don't underestimate the difference these small changes can make in helping a bizarre sleep schedule feel that much more manageable.

THE TEAMWORK FIX:
ENLIST SLEEP SUPPORT

I'll never forget a conversation I once had with one of my overnight producers at ABC, Liz Sobel. She'd worked that shift for years, and as I struggled to navigate my weekend sleep, I was curious how she handled hers. She was nearly in tears as she explained how hard it was because her kids always criticized her by saying, "You sleep all the time!" Imagine how frustrating it is to be sleep-deprived because of how hard you're working for your family, only for them to criticize you and imply that you're lazy because you dare to sleep at all.

Then there are the inevitable events and activities daytime sleepers have to miss. Think it's tough telling someone you can't go to an event because you have to go to work? Try telling them you can't go because you have to go to bed. Spoiler alert: It does not go over well, especially with children.

Shift work sleep consultant Carolyn Schur says this is why it's so important to have a family discussion about how you are going to deal with shift work—as a household. She suggests making sure the whole family knows when you're going to be sleeping and what that will mean for everyone else. Some questions she suggests include: How are we going to deal with childcare? How are we going to deal with all the household and domestic chores? How are we going to deal with activities we want to do? How are we going to deal with celebrations and holidays?

This may sound basic, but I wish someone had told me this when I first signed up to overnight hours. I hate missing out on things, and I really hate disappointing people, so when I started working the graveyard shift I continued my usual pattern of saying yes. Yes to every work assignment, every family event, every friend event, and every time my husband wanted to do something.

When my sleep fell apart, all this people-pleasing and FOMO blew up in my face. I ended up spending up to twelve hours a day in bed, trying to eke out whatever sleep I could get in dribs and drabs. After all that time in bed, I still felt like crap. Whatever energy I had I used to "turn it on" in front of the cameras. By the time I got home, I was spent. I'll never forget the day my husband confessed he was jealous of my co-anchor, Kendis Gibson, and my other colleagues. "They get the fun Diane," he said sadly.

Once I revised my sleep schedule, I started being more disciplined about saying no to activities that fell during my sleep window, so I could actually be well rested and present for those that fell during my wakeful hours. But I still felt a huge amount of guilt every single time I had to turn down an invitation. It all would have been so much easier had I just managed everyone else's—and my—expectations from the very beginning.

I'll also add to Schur's advice that if you have a job like mine, where you can get called in at any time, make sure to have that conversation with your supervisor as well. It took me reaching a breaking point before I finally worked up the courage to tell my boss just how much I was struggling. By the time I made it into her office, I was practically in tears—in fact I might have been actually in tears. I pride myself on being a hard worker, a team player, and a "yes" person, but constantly being asked to do things at all hours of the day took its toll, both physically and emotionally. I felt like I was being taken advantage of. I would often ask myself questions like, *They wouldn't ask someone else to do a standby shift in the middle of the night, so why are they asking me to do it in the middle of the day? They know I'm supposed to be sleeping!* Keep in mind, these kinds of scenarios can feel *way* more dramatic when you're sleep-deprived.

But my boss set off a lightbulb moment for me with a simple

question. "Does everyone know when you sleep?" she asked me. I was immediately annoyed, thinking, *Obviously they know when I sleep.* But as I went to answer her, I suddenly realized . . . that they didn't. For some reason it hadn't dawned on me that since different people on the night shift sleep at different times, no one actually knew which part of the day I was using for sleep.

We decided that 9:00 A.M. to 3:00 P.M. would be considered my "Do Not Disturb" window, barring breaking news. This allowed me to still be available for early morning shoots and late afternoon shoots, and guaranteed that on the very rare chance they both happened on the same day, I could still get roughly six hours in bed. More importantly, it ensured that my circadian rhythm could finally entrain to a consistent sleep window. Finally—and for me this was a big one—it meant I was no longer plagued with the emotional burden of having to choose between work and sleep all the time. I was no longer, or at least very rarely, put in that position. Instead, those who wanted me on a shoot would just schedule it around my sleep window.

So even if, like me, you're not willing to leave your job, it's worth having a talk with your boss and others involved in your everyday life to see if there might be small ways they can help you create a better sleep setup. You'd be surprised how even small changes can make a big difference, and you'd be surprised how willing some people are to work with you if you just ask.

THE EATING FIX:
MEAL PLAN

When and what to eat became a running joke during my time as a graveyard shifter. "How's dinner . . . or is it breakfast?" someone might ask if they saw you munching on something. The truth is, I usually had no idea. One day I'd eat a steak at 4:00 A.M.; another day it would be an egg sandwich. It's "brinner" time!

As I entrained my circadian rhythm, it became helpful to eat my meals according to my sleep schedule, just as Janine and Andrea did. My "breakfast" was in the evening as my husband ate dinner; "lunch" was at the beginning of my shift, around 11:00 P.M.; "dinner" was around 3:00 A.M.; and then I had my pre-bed snack around 8:00 A.M.

For those who haven't entrained their circadian rhythm, Carolyn Schur says, you'll find it helpful to instead eat two or three small meals throughout the night. "The digestive system was not designed to consume food at night. So if you go to standard three meals at night, you are going to have digestive problems," she tells me. To get around this, she suggests eating small amounts every two or three hours and choosing protein, "because protein-based foods metabolize more slowly, and that allows you to keep your blood sugar more stable and allows you to feel more satiated for longer periods of time."

Of course, the other obstacle to eating well during overnight hours is the limited access to healthy food—or in some cases, any food. There aren't many places delivering kale salads at 3:00 A.M. (not that I would have ordered them anyway . . . but that's not the point).

Eventually I started making my own make-ahead meals that were easy to microwave at the office. For more portable options, Schur suggests cheese and crackers, nuts, a hard-boiled egg, a banana, a package of tuna, yogurt, or if you're really short on time, an occasional chocolate milk, because it has protein, a little sugar, and a little caffeine. She says by keeping portable protein sources handy at work, "you know you always have a good nutritious source of food."

Still, Schur says those sleeping in opposition to their circadian rhythm have one more food challenge once they get home and go to bed: "our body is supposed to get nutrients during the day, and digest those nutrients, so they'll often wake up feeling hungry."

This is a classic example of when the common "don't eat three hours before bed" advice can lead you astray. Instead, Schur recommends a small snack of complex carbohydrates before bed, like whole wheat toast with peanut butter or some oatmeal with a little warm milk. Not only will this help stave off hunger, but complex carbs also have their own sleep-promoting benefits (more on that in chapter 19).

Also, see chapter 11 for more on how to strategically use fasting or time-restricted eating to cope with shift work.

THE ADVOCATE FIX:
BEWARE OF UNDIAGNOSED SLEEP DISORDERS

As a shift worker, it's easy to assume that if you're having sleep problems, it's got to be because of your work schedule. It's also easy for your doctor to make that same assumption, and unfortunately both of you may be wrong.

Schur says she's worked with countless shift workers who were surprised to learn they had undiagnosed sleep disorders like sleep apnea, insomnia, or restless legs syndrome. Many had the same experience I had: you go to the doctor, complain you can't sleep, tell them you're a shift worker, and the conversation stops there. They prescribe a sleeping pill and send you on your way.

Schur's advice: If you're doing everything you can to care for yourself and your sleep, and you still don't feel well-rested, be persistent with your physician and say, "I really think I need to be checked for a sleep disorder."

THE FORMAT FIX:
SHIFT WORK SLEEP DIARY

If you work the graveyard shift, trying to use a traditional sleep diary can feel like trying to fit into your favorite jeans from high school—it ain't happenin'.

Most sleep diaries follow the format of the Consensus Sleep Diary, with a list of questions on the left side and then seven columns in which to provide answers, one for each day of the week.

But Dr. Annie Vallières, a researcher at the Cervo Brain Research Centre in Quebec, says once she started studying shift workers, she realized there was a problem. "Shift workers sleep during the day, they nap, and they still sleep at night when they're not working at night. So that complexifies the evaluation of sleep," she tells me. She says when her patients would try to use the regular weekly sleep diary, they would fill it up in three days because they'd use one column for daytime sleep, another for evening sleep, and another if they took a short nap.

Vallières and her team are now working to validate a special shift work sleep diary, but in the meantime consider using a "two-week sleep diary," which has a space for each hour of the day instead of each day of the week. The one I've created below is based on a sleep diary from the Railroaders' Guide to Healthy Sleep and is made especially for graveyard shifters. For a version you can download and print, go to sleepfixbook.com.

No matter what diary you use, Vallières says, the most important part for shift workers is to record all sleep periods—daytime sleep, evening sleep, overnight nap, etc. Because even shift workers who are satisfied with their sleep tend to get it in at least two different shifts, but if you only record daytime sleep, on paper it will still appear that you're sleep-deprived.

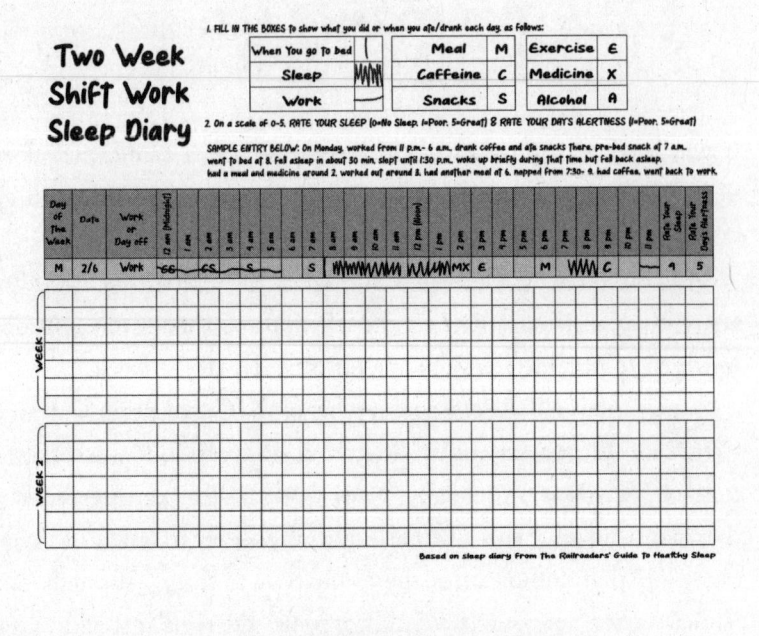

Based on sleep diary from The Railroaders' Guide To Healthy Sleep

THE ADJUSTED FIX:
STIMULUS CONTROL FOR SHIFT WORKERS

Like any insomniac, shift workers with insomnia need to reduce their time awake in bed, but those trying stimulus control, sleep restriction, or sleep compression should consider a few adjustments.

You might remember from chapter 5, a key component of these methods is the instruction that, if at any point you're awake long enough for it to bother you, get out of bed, do something relaxing, and return to bed when you feel sleepy. But Dr. Vallières says for daytime sleepers, their bedroom is often the only room that is dark during their sleep hours. Considering their circadian rhythm is naturally high at this time, if they leave that dark room, they may not feel genuinely sleepy for the rest of the day.

Then on weekends, when many shift back to sleeping at night, they're so used to working at night that they also might not get that feeling of genuine sleepiness if they're following traditional stimulus control rules overnight.

Instead, Vallières tells shift workers to get out of bed but stay in the dark, do something relaxing for five to ten minutes, then go back to bed. When I asked her what to do during these five to ten minutes, she suggested breathing exercises or even just walking around the room. You can also check out chapter 3 and 20 for other suggestions. I'd probably listen to a short podcast even if that meant going a little longer than ten minutes.

If you're staying in your room, it might also be helpful to have a comfortable chair to sit in. If your bed is the only option, try sitting on top of the covers, and on a different side from where you normally sleep. Anything to differentiate this time from when you're lying in bed to sleep.

Since I wasn't aware of these suggestions at the time, I did leave my room while practicing stimulus control during the day. And while my living room is not nearly as dark as my bedroom, I put the shades down and wore dark wraparound sunglasses to minimize my light exposure. Just another sign that you don't have to do these things perfectly for them to work—just find a way to make them work for you!

THE MISCOMMUNICATION FIX:
SHIFT WORK SLEEPING PILLS

Many shift workers face the challenge of sleeping during the day by turning to sleeping pills. But Dr. Vallières says too many are taking those pills at the wrong time, which can end up making you feel worse. That's because sleeping pills generally work best when taken at the same time of day. But Vallières says if a doctor tells a shift worker to take a sleeping pill thirty minutes before bed, they might take the pill in the morning before their first sleep period, then again before their evening nap. She says when the weekend hits and they switch to sleeping at night, they'll likely take a pill then too.

So, as I said earlier in the book, if you're taking sleeping pills regularly it should be under the guidance of a sleep specialist. Even then, make sure to clarify your schedule and establish a real plan for when you should be taking those pills.

If you're a doctor, Vallières says be sure to make your instructions extra clear when dealing with shift workers. "I think it would be important to tell them 'thirty minutes before going to bed *in the morning*,' for example, because if it's just 'thirty minutes before going to bed' and the person is going to bed three times in twenty-four hours . . . some will take it three times."

THE ROTATING FIX:
CLOCKWISE, QUICK, OR CONSISTENT

It is generally easier to delay than advance circadian rhythms, so if you are a rotating shift worker with any say in your schedule, aim for clockwise rotations, where you progressively start later in the day, rather than earlier. It's easier to go from day shift to evening shift to night shift, rather than night shift to evening shift to day shift.

Sleep experts also recommend that rotating schedules change quickly—two- to three-night shifts max—or stay unchanged for at least three weeks at a time. No medium rotations.

For quick rotations, the American Academy of Sleep Medicine also recommends limiting "shift duration to eight hours," allowing for "three days of recuperation after night shifts," and having the new shift start and end with at least one day off so you can adjust.

THE PRESCRIPTION FIX:
MODAFINIL

While shift workers notoriously love caffeine, it may be helpful to know caffeine isn't our only option to promote wakefulness. Modafinil and its sister drug armodafinil are actually FDA approved to reduce sleepiness associated with shift work. When I started asking sleep experts about these drugs, I expected to get negative feedback. But to my surprise, Dr. Chris Winter instead told me modafinil is a "godsend" for patients with both shift work disorder and insomnia.

I was skeptical, but as he continued to explain, it started to make sense. Winter says with modafinil, instead of telling patients, "Here's a drug to knock you out," he can tell them to go to bed at their established bedtime and "if you sleep, great! If you don't, it's okay. Take this drug. It'll make you feel like a million bucks."

This might sound like horrible advice. But Winter says the common joke about modafinil for insomnia is that "you take it once, you never take it again," because, ironically, by making insomniacs feel it's okay if they don't sleep, you remove the fear that's keeping them awake. In his experience, Winter says the drug also doesn't prevent patients from sleeping at bedtime the same way poorly timed caffeine does, another reason he often recommends modafinil to shift workers who struggle with their drive home.

Still, like any drug, modafinil can have side effects. Ginger Zee tells me that when she started taking it for narcolepsy, she felt amazing, productive, and after a month or two, she started feeling heightened emotions for the first time. "I was crying at movies. I had never cried at movies," she tells me. "I was excited about projects that I hadn't been excited about before . . . and it was really cool—until the fall."

While she was feeling more and more up during the day, Ginger says she started feeling more and more down at night as the drug wore off. She says, "That did not help my depression, and that's when I started having extreme bouts. So much so that I had my first suicide attempt very soon after."

Despite that, Ginger says she doesn't think the drug is bad—and she still stayed on it for fifteen years. But she wishes someone had given her a heads-up that it could have psychological effects, so she would have known to look out for them. Winter says, "With any medication that has central nervous system effects, even antidepressants, you need to be careful about mood changes."

This is yet another reason to be sure you're taking this or any sleep-related medication under the guidance of a sleep specialist and be sure to ask lots of questions about potential side effects. Winter also adds that it's best to use these drugs as a temporary solution to help you after a bad night or to help you while you work on a more permanent, drug-free solution to your sleep issues. Because while modafinil and armodafinil may help you feel awake, just like caffeine, they are not a replacement for sleep.

PART 4

SLEEP HABITS

The only thing more annoying than a list of things you have to do is a list of things you have to NOT do. That's often what articles on good sleep habits feel like: don't drink alcohol, don't have caffeine, don't eat too late, don't look at screens . . . the list goes on and on.

In a vacuum, with no other factors to consider, these would generally be sound pieces of sleep advice. But we don't live in a vacuum, and in the real world these things can also have consequences that have to be weighed against their benefits—especially if you have insomnia.

Even the list itself can have consequences. For starters, highlighting a bunch of dos and don'ts to improve sleep creates the impression that sleep is fragile, attainable only if we stick to a strict set of rules and patterns. It also creates the impression that perfect sleep habits will fix problems like insomnia. Some articles even outright state that. These false beliefs can make our problems worse, as can the frustration that comes with working really hard to perfect our sleep habits, only to find we are still sleeping like crap anyway.

These lists can also foster an all-or-nothing approach. You might decide you're not willing to make all these changes, so you just accept sleep problems as a necessary evil. It doesn't have to be this way.

Instead, as explained in chapter 2, think of sleep hygiene the same way you think of dental hygiene. It's good for improving dental health on the margins and to help prevent future problems, but if you already have a cavity, brushing and flossing obsessively is not going to fix the problem. In the same way, if your problems have been around for a while, sleep hygiene is unlikely to fix them, and obsessing over sleep hygiene will likely make your problems worse.

Common sense can go a long way here. If you're drinking a double espresso every evening and having trouble sleeping, changing that habit might have a significant impact on your sleep. If your sleep troubles started right around the same time you started playing video games at night, your troubleshooting should start there. But if there's no reason to suspect your sleep habits are what caused your sleep problem, there's no reason to believe perfecting your sleep habits will fix it.

Still, some habits do affect our sleep in less obvious ways. For example, caffeine can come from surprising sources, and can be more or less effective depending on a long list of factors. Screens, for all the bad press they get, can sometimes indirectly *help* our sleep. And alcohol, despite being the world's most popular sleep aid, is actually terrible for sleep.

So use parts 1 through 3 of this book to try to identify and address the underlying cause of what's keeping you awake. Then use parts 4 and 5 to get a full, nuanced explanation for how certain aspects of sleep habits and environment affect our sleep so you can decide what changes make the most sense for you.

CHAPTER 15

Booze and Snooze

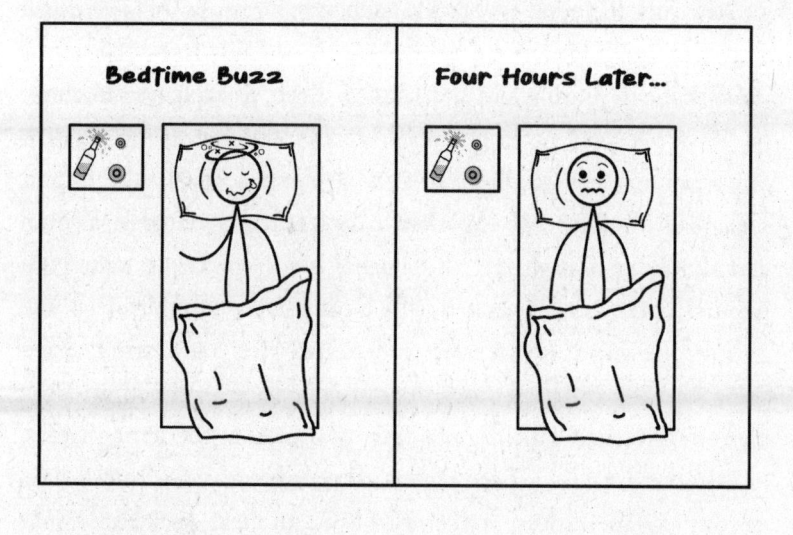

Bedtime Buzz · Four Hours Later...

NOT A DAY PASSES THAT I don't see an ad for some new drug or device claiming it can help me sleep (target marketing is on to me). But despite this booming industry, the most commonly used sleep aid is still an old favorite: alcohol.

According to the Sleep Foundation, "as many as 20 percent of Americans use alcohol to help them fall asleep." It's easy to see why: booze does help you fall asleep. Drink enough, and it can even make you pass out. For those with sleep problems, this can be especially tempting.

I can recall the many times I would have "one more drink" during our occasional early morning happy hour—for the sole purpose of getting that extra push to pass out once I got home from the night shift. And it would work . . . kind of. On those days I would get in bed, put my head on the pillow, and within minutes I was out. It was such a nice contrast to my usual routine of lying in bed awake and frustrated. But despite the popularity of the nightcap, alcohol is a terrible sleep aid, as I would come to learn a few hours later.

For starters, alcohol helps us fall asleep by boosting adenosine and relaxing our muscles, but the adenosine boost is short-lived, and that muscle relaxation also affects the throat muscles—making us more prone to snoring and sleep apnea. Then, as explained in chapter 10, as we sober up in our sleep, alcohol withdrawal messes with our body temperature rhythm, as well as our cortisol rhythm and melatonin rhythm. For those with restless legs syndrome, alcohol can also make that worse. And alcohol is a diuretic—it makes you pee and leaves you dehydrated, which can each wreck your sleep too.

So while we might fall asleep more easily after a few drinks, staying asleep is a different story. As our adenosine level comes down and our circadian wake signals start to fire off at the wrong times, our sleep is disrupted. Even more so if your breathing is interrupted or your legs are restless. For some, this might mean very brief awakenings that you're not aware of, but that wreck the quality of your sleep. For others, like me, within a few hours you're wide awake, heart racing, dehydrated, and unable to get back to sleep—despite feeling exhausted.

In an extra-cruel twist, Dr. Timothy Roehrs says his research shows someone with severe insomnia may not experience the negative effect on sleep right away. "When these people drink alcohol, their sleep is normalized," he tells me. After a low dose of alcohol right before bed, "they fall asleep quickly, and they actually stay asleep the whole night." But Roehrs, the director of research at the Sleep Disorders and Research Center of Henry Ford Health System, says after just three nights, insomniacs develop a tolerance to those initial sedating effects and the alcohol starts to disturb their sleep.

The common response to this? Drink more the next night. Roehrs says, "This is the trap of alcohol."

But here's the strangest part about my own experience. Though that drunken sleep I used to get after happy hour was low quality and short lived, I still felt grateful for that respite of easy sleep. It was sleep I didn't have to think or worry about. Healthy sleepers may have a hard time understanding this, but with alcohol, I had sleep confidence, and in many ways the hangover felt worth it.

Thankfully, my drinking was limited to social events. I never got into the habit of coming home and pouring myself a nightcap (or more accurately, a daycap). But for those who do, this is not me judging. This is me telling you I totally get it, and there is a better way.

While this is usually the part where the author explains that this is why they don't drink anymore and you shouldn't either, for this author, that would be a lie. I do still enjoy an occasional cocktail or two, but I no longer use alcohol to help me sleep. On the contrary, I've learned a few ways to limit alcohol's effect on my sleep instead.

THE CURFEW FIX:
CUT YOURSELF OFF

By far the most effective way to limit alcohol's effect on sleep is to cut yourself off early enough to sober up before bedtime. On average it takes about an hour to process a shot, beer, cocktail, or glass of wine, so Roehrs says a good rule of thumb is if you're having one drink, finish it at least an hour before bed, and if you're having multiple drinks, finish them two to three hours before bed. As to whether you should give yourself time to sober up even if it means going to bed later, Roehrs says it's not clear, but it is possible that "if you stay awake for another hour and then try to sleep, then maybe you would sleep better."

THE DUAL PURPOSE FIX:
FOOD

You may have heard that food helps you sober up by "soaking up" the alcohol you've consumed. I'm sorry to report that this is not true. But while eating *after* drinking won't do much to sober you up, food before or with alcohol can offer dual benefits.

For one, a full stomach slows the absorption of alcohol into the bloodstream. This isn't so much because the food absorbs the alcohol, but more because our stomach absorbs alcohol much more slowly than our intestine does. When we drink liquids, they basically pass right through to the intestine. But food needs to be processed by the stomach first. Thus drinking on a full stomach will keep the alcohol in the stomach longer, where it will be absorbed more slowly, giving your liver more time to process it.

Another benefit of food is that it boosts the liver's ability to process alcohol. As Dr. Marie-Pierre St-Onge explains, "The amount of the enzyme in the liver that detoxifies alcohol is greater in the fed state than the fasted state." Thus food can indirectly help the liver process and eliminate alcohol faster.

As for what kind of food to eat, according to a 2012 study, "meals high in either fat, or carbohydrate or protein are equally effective," both in slowing down gastric emptying and in increasing the alcohol metabolic rate—aka how quickly alcohol is eliminated from your system.

Of course even on a full stomach, drinking a lot will still overwhelm your liver and spike your blood alcohol level, so enjoy in moderation.

THE ALTERNATING FIX:
HYDRATION

Water is another multipurpose tool to lessen the effects of alcohol on sleep. Consuming an adequate amount of water not only helps combat dehydration but also, as Dr. Roehrs points out, "the additional water might help you clear the alcohol from your system, because you're urinating." But unlike we used to do in college, Roehrs says this does not mean you should chug massive amounts of water right before bed. Otherwise, you'll have to wake up to pee.

Instead, several experts I spoke to suggest alternating a glass of water or something with electrolytes in it, between each alcoholic drink. As an added bonus, that time spent drinking water is time spent not drinking alcohol.

THE THINK AHEAD FIX:
PREP YOUR SLEEP ENVIRONMENT

In addition to the many issues listed above, alcohol lowers our arousal threshold later in the night, meaning we are awoken more easily by sleep disruptions. So a light, sound, or temperature change that we might normally sleep through will suddenly be enough to wake us up. You can help counter this by ensuring your sleep environment is as conducive to sleep and as disruption proof as possible. See part 5 for more on that.

It's also best to prep your bedroom *before* you go out drinking.

If you don't feel like searching for your sleep mask or setting up your sound machine now, you're *definitely* not going to after three cocktails.

THE DON'T MIX FIX:
NO SLEEP MEDS

Taking a sleeping pill might sound like the easiest way to counter alcohol's sleep-disrupting properties but to put it mildly, sleeping pills and alcohol do not mix. As clinical psychologist Dr. Michael Breus explains on his blog thesleepdoctor.com, sleeping pills can actually multiply alcohol's effects. Not only can this harm your sleep, but Breus also notes, "many of the weird behaviors reported on sleeping pills is when they are mixed with alcohol. It is dangerous and should always be avoided."

THE KILLJOY FIX:
DRINKING "IN MODERATION"

People often talk about drinking "in moderation" as a general term, but did you know there's an actual amount associated with that? The *2015–2020 Dietary Guidelines for Americans* defines moderate drinking as up to two drinks per day for men and one drink per day for women. But to minimize sleep disruption, you still can't have those drinks too close to bedtime. And no, unfortunately it's not the same thing if you "save up" and have all those drinks on the weekend instead.

THE SEE FOR YOURSELF FIX:
BOOZE BREAK

Read all you want about alcohol's impact on sleep, the best way to understand how it impacts *your* sleep is to spend some time without it. Neurologist and sleep specialist Dr. Chris Winter advises giving up all alcohol for two weeks. After those two weeks, you can evaluate how you feel and decide for yourself if it's worth ditching your dinner wine.

CHAPTER 16

The Truth About Screens

STOP ME IF YOU'VE HEARD this one before: screens emit blue light, which is terrible for sleep, thus you should swear off all screens at least two hours before bed . . . and don't even *think* about bringing that phone into the bedroom.

You'll be hard-pressed to find a sleep article that doesn't have some variation of this warning. But while the logic sounds very straightforward, the reality is much more nuanced.

The Rabbit Hole

Dr. Michael Grandner says that while talking about blue light sounds very compelling and scientific, he believes the bigger problem with screens near bedtime is a mental engagement that depends largely on what you're using the screens for. He and his team examined this in a 2015 study, comparing how 1,000 survey respondents used devices before bedtime with how they slept. Having the device in the room showed no correlation with sleep issues. Neither did certain behaviors, like texts and phone calls. But nightly emailing and browsing the internet were associated with issues like insomnia and short sleep. Grandner explains, "If you were doing something that was a little more mentally engaging, then you were more likely to have disrupted sleep." A 2013 study of device use within an hour of bedtime found similar results: the more interactive a device was, the more likely it was that the person using it would have difficulty falling asleep and unrefreshing sleep.

To add to this problem, Grandner says, content is now engineered to be continually reinforcing. We can endlessly scroll through social media feeds, video games can last upwards of thirty hours, even our TV shows are continuous—in some cases the next episode starts automatically.

This all makes it that much harder to disengage and that much easier to lose track of time and our own sleepiness. The next thing you know, it's hours later and you're not just still awake, you're too revved up to sleep well.

I often fell into this trap while trying to do something time-sensitive before bed, like put in a grocery order. Usually I would first try to convince myself to skip it altogether, telling myself the groceries can wait—we'll eat takeout. But inevitably I'd end up with the grocery list swirling around in my head. So I'd throw in the towel and pick up my phone. But before pulling up my grocery app, I'd decide to quickly check my email. *"Ooh, an Amazon order shipped. Let me see which one!"* So I go to Amazon, but before I check my orders, a vanity mirror in the product suggestions catches my eye. *I have been meaning to build a mini vanity in the bedroom. I wonder if they have a small gold mirror?* I search through a few and don't find quite what I'm looking for. But I remember seeing a good one in a hairstyle tutorial video not too long ago. So I go to YouTube and *Oh no, don't do it! Don't get distracted by the animal videos. You know you always get sucked into the* . . . Click! *Ah! The dog's singing "Let It Go" That's hilarious! Ooh, there's one with a baby singing "Let It Go." How cute is that? WAIT, focus, Diane, vanity mirror, remember? Right, let's search "hair tutorial videos." Nope, not that one. Not that one, but I like that braid—let's save that. Ugh, I can't find this stupid video. But I bet Pinterest has some good ideas. So I go* over to Pinterest, where after cruising dozens of ridiculous DIYs, I see a post about using makeup to make eyes look more youthful. I want youthful eyes! So I click on the post, which is actually an ad for an eye brightener that claims to make you look like you've "had 9 hours of sleep last night." And then it hits me: *Sleep! I'm supposed to be sleeping!* But now that I've spent all this time futzing around the internet, I have no chance of getting seven hours, let alone nine. Oh, and also . . . I still have no groceries.

The Bright Side of Screens

While screen time can hinder sleep, it can also provide a frequently ignored benefit. Dr. James Wyatt, a researcher and clinician specializing in sleep disorders at Rush University, tells me, "A lot of patients will come in and they'll say, 'Oh, I've done all the things I know I should. I'm avoiding all TV for two hours before bed.' And I say, 'Well, that's absurd, you need to do something to wind down.'"

Wyatt says this is especially important for insomniacs because screen time often "helps them shut their mind off from their worries and concerns of the day." Remove all screens within an hour or two of bedtime, and Wyatt says, blue light might be reduced, but his bigger concern is "now they've got even more time to worry and ruminate."

This was indirectly communicated to me when I went to see an acupuncturist recommended by my fertility doctor. My husband and I had been trying to conceive for at least three years, and I couldn't help thinking my sleep was part of the problem. Suffice it to say, the added pressure didn't make sleeping any easier. When I sat down for my first appointment, the acupuncturist asked all sorts of questions about my job, my personal life, my schedule, my habits. And then she stumped me: "What do you do that's just for you?" she asked. I kept coming up with answers, but she kept ruling them out because they benefited my job, my husband, or some other third party. Finally I got it. "I watch *Real Housewives*!" I told her, "It doesn't help me as a journalist, my husband *hates* it—it's purely for my enjoyment." Her response: "Do more of that." So I made *Real Housewives* part of my "evening" ritual. Turns out it was much more soothing to fall asleep thinking about other people's drama, instead of my own.

So if you find a screen curfew helps you to relax at the end of the day, great! If you find you're more anxious without that screen time, or if you need to be on a screen for work, consider the tools below instead.

THE MIND-BLOWING FIX:
THE GRAYSCALE TRICK

My favorite hack to avoid getting sucked down a rabbit hole without giving up my phone is the grayscale trick: you set your device color filter to grayscale, turning everything on it black and white. Dr. Michael Grandner says he first learned this from a patient who used to spend hours in bed on her phone. "It was extremely effective for her and every other place I've deployed it," he tells me.

Our conversation was interestingly timed because we were in the thick of the Covid-19 pandemic, and being stuck at home feeling disconnected had me mindlessly scrolling social media much more than usual. I was so excited about Grandner's tip, I put my phone on grayscale immediately—right in the middle of our call. A week later I was shocked: my screen time was down 42 percent!

Each device is different, but this setting is usually somewhere in the Color Filters settings. I now have it set to a shortcut key. If I want to see something on the phone in color, I click three times. As soon as I'm done, I click three times again to reinstate grayscale.

The best part about this trick is the device still works exactly the same as before, so there's not much being sacrificed. If I remember I want to put in a grocery order before bed, I can still do that, no problem. But even if I decide to "quickly" check Instagram while I'm there, it really becomes a quick check, no more mindless scrolling. Something about black and white just makes it all less addictive—in my case, 42 percent less.

THE UPRIGHT FIX:
SCREEN TIME = STANDING TIME

Grandner's second tip to limit screen time before bed is more of a rule: "Instead of getting into bed with your phone, stand next to your bed with your phone. You can be on it, but you have to be standing." He says this eliminates the typical problem of getting sucked in and failing to notice signals like sleepiness. "If you're standing, you're not totally out of touch with your body," Grandner tells me. "Eventually . . . you're going to want to sit down, and your sitting down is your body telling you you're done. You don't need to relax anymore, you're ready."

I use a cheater's version of this rule with myself: I can look at my phone while I'm sitting in bed, but if I want to lie down, the phone has to go down too.

THE OUTSOURCE YOUR WILLPOWER FIX:
VICE APPS CURFEW

Before learning the grayscale trick, I implemented what I call a "vice apps" curfew. Rather than a screen curfew, this is a curfew for just the apps or websites that tend to distract and suck you in.

You can do this either by disabling certain apps after a certain time of day or by placing daily limits on how much you can use a particular app. Some devices have this ability built in, or you can choose from a number of third-party apps that will do this across multiple platforms and devices. They're usually marketed as "anti-distraction" apps aimed at helping productivity, but limiting those distractions can also help you get to bed and go to sleep.

THE LAZY FIX:
PASSIVE ACTIVITY

When using screens to unwind, opt for more passive activities whenever possible, where you are an observer rather than a participant. Watching a movie or show, for example, is preferable to playing a video game or perusing social media. TV shows and movies also have the added bonus of having a clear end.

If you're a sucker for Netflix's autoplay feature, consider disabling it. This means at the end of each episode, you'll have to choose to keep watching, rather than choose to turn it off, which can make all the difference when you're considering "just one more."

THE BRIGHTNESS FIX:
DIM/DARK MODE

To limit the impact of evening light from your screens, start by limiting their brightness, which you'll actually need very little of if you've reduced the light in your surroundings, as advised in chapter 8. On computer monitors, brightness adjustments might be on the monitor itself, in the computer settings, or both. For phones and tablets, you can do this in settings, and many also have shortcut commands. Lowering the contrast can also help reduce the intensity of your screen light.

There are also a few ways to limit brightness even further than standard settings permit:

Dark Mode/Dark Theme

Dark mode or dark theme essentially transforms light backgrounds with dark text into black backgrounds with light text. This not only reduces light exposure to the eye but can also help save on battery life. Most mobile devices and computers now have this as a stand-alone option in the display settings and/or as a color filter. It may also be called something like "inverted," "reverse polarity," or "negative colors."

I set my phone to do this automatically every evening, then go back to normal in the morning. You can also create a shortcut, to easily turn it on and off at will.

Extra Dim

Just because your brightness is turned all the way down doesn't mean your screen can't be any dimmer. iPhones, for example, have a little-known low light option hidden as a zoom filter in the zoom settings (Google "how to get low light on iPhone" for more detailed instructions). Add that to your accessibility shortcuts and you can make your phone extra dim just by triple clicking the side button. Third-party apps also offer extra-dim options for both phones and computers.

THE WARM IT UP FIX:
CHANGE COLOR TONE

In addition to reducing how bright your screens are, you can also limit their negative impact on sleep by reducing how blue or "cool" they are. There's little data on the effects of blue-light-blocking software, but many doctors I've spoken to recommend it, and a 2019 study on night shift workers did find using the blue-light-blocking software f.lux on their computers improved the quality of their sleep and left them feeling less drowsy during their shift.

Many phones and even newer TVs now offer similar technology, like Apple's Night Shift mode. For any that don't, third-party apps are available for phones and add-on products like driftTV are available for your television.

This is yet another thing my phone and computer do automatically every evening. I haven't made any adjustments to my TV, but as you'll see from the next Fix, I'm not too concerned about that.

For a more low-tech and universal option, you can also try blue-light-blocking glasses. A 2018 study found that fourteen insomniacs slept significantly longer and better after wearing amber-tinted blue-light-blocking glasses two hours before bed for a week.

Just make sure you're not using these features all day long, because while blue light gets a bad rap, blue light during the day is actually good for your circadian rhythm. So to help sleep, use these features only in the hours leading up to your bedtime.

THE BACK IT UP FIX:
SCREEN DISTANCE

Remember when your parents used to warn you about sitting too close to the TV? Yet another way Mama really did know best. Since distance from a light source reduces the amount of light hitting the eye, the farther away you are from a screen, the better. So, counterintuitively, it's often preferable to watch movies or shows on a television rather than on a computer or tablet. While it's true the TV screen is bigger, the fact that you're sitting farther away means less light is getting to your eye.

That said, TVs are getting brighter and brighter, so consider lowering the brightness and/or wearing sunglasses if yours seems particularly bright. If you do watch on a phone or tablet, turn the brightness down and consider propping it up rather than holding it, so you can sit farther away.

CHAPTER 17

Caffeine All Wrong

THE CONVERSATION AROUND CAFFEINE AND sleep is usually a short one: caffeine is bad for your sleep, so to sleep better, avoid it. The end. But if you have sleep problems and you're still consuming caffeine, I'm guessing it's not because no one ever told you it can disrupt your sleep. It's probably because quitting caffeine is hard—*especially* when you're having sleep issues. And, if caffeine can help you stick with a consistent wake time after a bad night, quitting caffeine may not even be advisable when initially addressing your sleep problems.

So instead of convincing you to quit caffeine, let's talk about how to maximize its benefits and minimize its negative effects. Because the truth is, most of us are doing caffeine all wrong.

THE HEAR ME OUT FIX:
HAVE CAFFEINE LATER

Despite what marketers would like us to believe, "the best part of waking up" should not be a cup of coffee. To understand why, you have to understand how caffeine actually works.

Caffeine's main function is to block adenosine, the chemical in the brain that makes us feel sleepy. You might remember from chapter 5 that adenosine accumulates when we're awake and dissipates while we sleep. So when we wake up in the morning, our adenosine level is at its lowest. Yet, when do most people consume caffeine? First thing in the morning, when there's little to no adenosine for the caffeine to block. This is a waste.

Another function of caffeine is to boost cortisol. But for most people, cortisol peaks within an hour of waking up, so if you're having coffee first thing in the morning, your cortisol levels are already high. Again, this is a waste. As Dr. Michael Breus puts it, "coffee in the morning is like throwing water on an already extinguished fire."

You might be thinking, *Then why do I feel energized after my morning cup of coffee?* If you consume caffeine daily, what you're feeling is likely the reversal of your caffeine withdrawal. That means the caffeine isn't "giving you energy," it's just getting you back to baseline. Breus says we're also likely feeling the adrenaline hit that caffeine provides. But because our cortisol levels are already up, this doesn't make us feel more awake—it makes us jittery.

Sleep Inertia

There is one more reason people may feel more awake after their morning coffee: sleep inertia. The idea that people who are well rested should jump out of bed full of energy is a myth. Most of us experience some form of sleep inertia, a period of grogginess that comes as the brain transitions from a sleep state to a wakeful state. Sleep inertia has been shown to last anywhere from 1 minute to 4 hours, but unless you're badly sleep-deprived, it's usually gone within 30 minutes. So, many of us might think it's the coffee getting us out of our morning fog, when actually it's just our brain naturally awakening on its own.

But while your ritual morning coffee may not do much to wake you up, it does have one significant effect: it raises your caffeine tolerance.

Dr. James Wyatt suggests that "a rational strategy for caffeine would be none in the morning and a minimal dose around, let's say, lunchtime, so in the middle of one's day." If that sounds too late for you, Dr. Michael Breus suggests waiting at least 90 minutes after waking up to have coffee and having water and sunlight first thing in the morning instead. If you just can't do without the ritual of your morning coffee, try switching that early cup to decaf. See the section below on tapering techniques for more on that.

THE FLIP-SIDE FIX:
. . . BUT NOT TOO LATE

I know, I know. I just told you to drink caffeine later, but we all know that having caffeine too late can disrupt our sleep. So how late is too late?

The most common guideline is to avoid caffeine within six hours of bedtime, but how long caffeine stays in the system varies widely from person to person. As Dr. Wyatt explains, "It's bizarre, that the half-life can vary between three and seven hours. That's a huge difference!"

To be clear, that doesn't mean that it takes three to seven hours for caffeine to leave your system, it means it takes three to seven hours for *half* of the caffeine you've consumed to leave your system. Then another three to seven hours for *half* of the remaining caffeine to leave your system, and so on.

To complicate things, caffeine half-life can also be affected by external factors. Smoking shortens it, by up to 50 percent. But liver disease, cytochrome inhibitors, and steroidal hormones prolong it. That last part is especially important for women, because oral contraceptives tend to double caffeine half-life. Still, it seems nothing impacts caffeine metabolism more than pregnancy, which on average extends half-life by more than eight hours, and in some cases adds up to sixteen hours to your usual caffeine half-life.

For those who metabolize slowly, that means even if you keep the recommended caffeine curfew of six hours before bed, you'll still have more than half of the caffeine you consumed in your system as you're trying to sleep. You might even have nearly *all* of it still in your system. Depending on how much you consume and how caffeine-sensitive you are, that can be more than enough to significantly disturb your sleep. The worst part is, you might not even know it.

A 2013 study showed 400 milligrams of caffeine six hours before bed "reduced sleep by more than 1 hour" compared to placebo. Granted, that's about four cups of regular coffee—more caffeine than most Americans drink in a day. But what I find most interesting is that, even after all that caffeine, and after objective monitors showed they lost more than an hour of sleep, the participants didn't note any sleep disturbance in their diaries.

The study's lead author, Dr. Christopher Drake of the Henry Ford Health System, tells me, "It's mostly that their sleep was fragmented. You're just waking up for a few minutes here and there and you really don't recognize it. You wake up in the morning thinking you had a decent amount of sleep."

Caffeine Circadian Effects

In addition to interfering with our sleep due to its alerting properties, late consumption of caffeine can also interfere with our circadian rhythm. A 2016 study demonstrated this by giving five participants the equivalent of a double espresso three hours before their usual bedtime. The researchers found the caffeine delayed subjects' melatonin rhythms by an average of forty minutes—roughly half the delay they saw with three hours of bright light therapy. "So it's not just sleep/wake states, but it's also affecting the fundamental clock mechanism," the study's coauthor, Dr. Ken Wright, tells me.

That means an occasional after-dinner coffee won't just keep you up late tonight, it will make you want to wake up later the next morning and stay up later the next night too. As the study's coauthor Dr. John O'Neill puts it: "You'll feel jet-lagged." All of these effects can then become compounded into what's called the caffeine loop: you get poor sleep due to caffeine, so the next day you compensate . . . with more caffeine, which leads to more poor sleep. Rinse. Repeat.

So if you suspect your caffeine might be impacting your sleep, try cutting yourself off earlier than you normally do and see how that works for you. But don't just look at how you think you slept—look at how you feel the following day or two, because we don't all notice when our sleep is interrupted, but we all know when we feel like crap.

If you own a sleep tracker, you can also use that to see if it records any noticeable difference in your sleep with different caffeine timing. But keep in mind sleep trackers generally aren't great at recording sleep cycles or overall sleep and can offer confusing or inaccurate data at times, so use this only to make loose comparisons, not to overanalyze the intricacies of your sleep.

THE STRATEGIC FIX:
CAFFEINE VS. SLEEP INERTIA

While regular morning sleep inertia usually clears within 30 minutes, it tends to be more severe and long lasting if we're suddenly woken up out of deep sleep. This typically happens if you're woken up in the middle of the night or if you take a nap while sleep-deprived, since sleep deprivation leads us to go into deep sleep more quickly. This kind of sleep inertia doesn't just leave you a little groggy: it can leave you feeling downright drunk.

"Now, say that someone awakens in an emergency, such as a paramedic, firefighter, physician, security guard, a military person—now they've got to perform under those conditions," Dr. Ken Wright, director of the Sleep and Chronobiology Laboratory at the University of Colorado–Boulder, tells me. In cases like these, he says, caffeine can be useful, especially in a rapid delivery form like caffeine gum, which has been shown to get caffeine into the bloodstream faster than when consumed in liquid form.

But even with the help of caffeine, Dr. Wright says it's crucial to have other safeguards in place when sleep inertia is likely. "For example, the physician giving a certain medication and a certain dose to the nurse . . . Perhaps someone else needs to make that decision or at least this needs to be checked . . . because they may be making poor decisions."

THE COUNTERINTUITIVE FIX:
CAFFEINE NAP

The other area where sleep inertia can prove especially dangerous is on the road. We always hear that if we feel drowsy while driving, we should take a nap. But if you wake up with sleep inertia, then get back on the road—you're essentially driving drunk. Instead consider a caffeine nap. As Dr. Wright explains, "You can actually take caffeine before that nap at the rest stop. And then when you wake up, the caffeine has kicked in. And you're going to have very little sleep inertia because of that."

In this case, espresso is usually recommended, since you want to be able to consume the caffeine quickly, then get your nap in before the caffeine kicks in. If you're a "bad napper," like me, a caffeine pill will give you a little more time to fall asleep and squeeze in a power nap before the caffeine hits your bloodstream.

That said, as mentioned in chapter 5, forcing yourself to stay awake is a little like holding your breath—eventually the body takes over and takes a breath or a nap, no matter how hard you try to fight it. Your best bet if you're too drowsy to drive: Find a different way to get home. As someone who lost a loved one very close to me due to drowsy driving, I promise you it's not worth the risk.

THE HATE TO BREAK IT TO YOU
FIX:
CAFFEINE RESET

According to the National Sleep Foundation, people "typically develop a strong tolerance to a daily dose of caffeine somewhere between a week and 12 days." Unfortunately, this tolerance can develop even faster if you're extremely sleep deprived. A 2016 study found that for participants limited to only five hours of sleep, the alerting and performance-enhancing effects of caffeine wore off after just three nights.

The good news for daily caffeine consumers is this means the same level of caffeine will affect your sleep less and less as you grow more tolerant. The bad news: You'll need more and more caffeine to get your desired effects in the daytime. The really bad news: You might also become dependent on caffeine, meaning if you don't have it, you experience withdrawal symptoms like headaches, irritability, and fatigue.

You can avoid this by having a routine caffeine reset. How frequent or long the break needs to be will depend on many factors, including how much caffeine you regularly consume. But you might, for example, take two days off every week, or one week off every month. This allows you to avoid the caffeine loop and maintain caffeine's efficacy, so it's there for you when you need it most.

THE GRADUAL FIX:
TAPERING TECHNIQUES

If you've already developed a caffeine tolerance and want to cut back or quit, you can minimize or avoid withdrawal symptoms by doing so gradually, also known as tapering.

How-To: Caffeine Tapering

One of the easiest ways to taper off caffeine is by finding a decaf version of your usual caffeinated drink, like decaf coffee, decaf tea, or decaf soda, as recommended by Dr. Michael Breus. Then follow his instructions below:

Week 1: Replace your usual caffeinated drink with ¼ decaf + ¾ regular.
Week 2: Up the ratio to half decaf + half regular.
Week 3: Up the ratio again to ¾ decaf + ¼ regular.
Week 4: If you're not ready to go full decaf, alternate between drinking all decaf, and ¾ decaf + ¼ regular mix, every other day.
Week 5: If you haven't already, switch to full decaf.

Dr. James Wyatt suggests another good general guideline is to reduce your caffeine by 50 mg every two days. Wyatt says, when it comes to caffeine tapering, "slow and steady typically wins the race."

Nutritionist Shawn Stevenson also suggests consuming more fiber as you taper. He writes in his book *Sleep Smarter,* "Having a temporary reduction in the gusto of your digestion is normal when you're breaking the coffee habit, but upping your fiber and water intake will help move things along (pun totally intended)."

THE AWARENESS FIX:
AVOID SURPRISING STIMULANTS

While the conversation around caffeine usually centers on coffee, caffeine comes in many different forms, and some of them may surprise you. "One 5-ounce bar of dark chocolate has the same amount of caffeine as a cup of coffee," Dr. Satchin Panda writes in his book *The Circadian Code.* You can also find caffeine in things like tea, certain medications, and even fitness drinks.

Dr. Chris Winter, who specializes in treating sleep issues in athletes, tells me he sees caffeine or similar stimulants popping up more and more in products meant to be consumed before or during exercise. "It's sort of infiltrated everything, and it is a performance-enhancing drug that needs to be used with a plan," he tells me.

Dr. James Wyatt says even coffee drinkers usually think only about how many cups of coffee they have and not how large those cups are and how strong that coffee is. "People just vastly underestimate the amount of caffeine that they have," he tells me.

So when trying to analyze how caffeine impacts you, don't forget to look beyond just how many cups of coffee you had. You may be consuming a lot more caffeine than you think.

THE CIRCADIAN FIX:
CAFFEINE PHASE DELAY

Just as caffeine can hinder circadian rhythm, it can also be used as a circadian tool, though it's one we know fairly little about. As mentioned above, occasional or "acute" evening caffeine has been shown to phase delay circadian rhythm in humans. But this works only if you haven't had caffeine in a while.

So if you want to try using caffeine to delay circadian rhythm, for a trip perhaps, make sure you don't have caffeine for roughly one to three days prior. You'll also want to ensure you have the amount and timing right. Wright recommends having roughly 200 milligrams of caffeine, roughly three to four hours before your usual bedtime in your original time zone.

This approach is not as effective as timed light exposure, but it's another tool to consider.

THE PERSPECTIVE FIX:
WORRY BEATS CAFFEINE

While caffeine can be disruptive to your sleep, it's important to keep its effects in perspective. Dr. Jason Ong says in the roughly fifteen years he's been treating patients, he can recall maybe two instances where caffeine intake was extreme enough that it needed to be addressed. This was a sentiment echoed by many of the specialists I spoke to.

So see the fixes above as ways to improve your sleep, not treatments to fix it. If you do have too much caffeine one day, the best thing you can do is carry on and try not to worry about it, because while most of us can still sleep with some caffeine in our system, you know what's way worse for our sleep? Worrying about caffeine.

CHAPTER 18

To Eat or Not to Eat

WHILE THE FINDINGS ON THE circadian effects of fasting are fairly new, the recommendation to have a large gap between your last meal and your bedtime is not. For years we've heard that to keep acid reflux from disturbing our sleep, we should stop eating two, three, or even four hours before going to bed. The logic makes sense: our stomach secretes acid to digest food, so lying down before we're done digesting makes it easier for that acid to travel up our esophagus, giving us acid reflux and heartburn.

But, as I touched on in chapter 11, this advice ignores the fact that some of us—like me—can't fall asleep or stay asleep if we go to bed hungry. As the Alaska Sleep Clinic explains on its website, sleeping on an empty stomach "can keep you mentally alert with hunger pains. This leads to an unsuccessful night's sleep." And guess what an unsuccessful night's sleep can cause? Acid reflux.

I learned this the hard way when I tried to improve my sleep by not eating within three hours of bedtime. My hunger made my sleep worse, which aggravated my acid reflux. But I didn't know it was the sleep deprivation that was making my reflux worse—so what did I do? I stopped eating even earlier. Which made me even more hungry, which made me sleep even less, which made my acid reflux even worse. It wasn't long before I gave up. I accepted acid reflux as inevitable and just started eating whenever I wanted to.

So what's the right answer? Don't eat close to bedtime or don't go to bed with an empty stomach?

You might remember from chapter 11 that chronic insomniacs experience elevated cortisol levels at night, likely due to conditioned arousal or circadian issues. And in the next chapter you'll learn about how carbs help lower cortisol. So it's possible that those with chronic insomnia or circadian rhythm disorders have a unique need for food closer to bedtime, at least until they can get their cortisol rhythms back on track.

A study from back in the eighties might also help shed some light on this. Researchers tested the effects of malted milk before bed by comparing it to having regular milk before bed and having a placebo capsule. What they found was that the results actually depended on the participants' usual eating habits. Those who usually ate a lot after 5:00 P.M. slept significantly better after drinking either milk. Those who usually ate a little after 5:00 P.M. slept better with the placebo capsule, which had no nourishment. Adding to that, the amount of benefit or impairment directly correlated with how much they usually ate near bedtime. The less a person usually ate near bedtime, the more their sleep was impaired by drinking either milk before bed. The more they usually ate near bedtime, the more their sleep was impaired by not having any nourishment before bed. The authors concluded that "a departure from a person's usual pattern of food intake in the evening impairs subsequent sleep."

So if you don't usually eat close to bedtime, even a supposed sleep-inducing snack may disturb your sleep. And if you are used to a nighttime snack, rather than eliminating it entirely—as so many recommend—you might be better off focusing on eating the right nighttime snack, at least to start. See more on that below.

THE ENJOYABLE FIX:
PRE-BED SNACK

When I set out to fix my insomnia, I didn't know about any of the science mentioned above, but I learned by trial and error that the "don't eat within three hours of bedtime" rule didn't work for me. So I decided to embrace another suggestion sometimes touted by sleep experts: eat a small snack an hour before bed to stave off hunger.

I also addressed the quantity and quality of the food I was eating. Instead of aiming to feel full, I started aiming to feel satisfied. So I swapped heavy meals for smaller, lighter choices that are still easy to prepare but less likely to trigger acid reflux. Typical options for me include a bowl of non-sugary cereal with almond milk (regular milk makes me clear my throat a lot), whole grain toast with butter or peanut butter, a cup of tomato-free soup (tomato triggers my acid reflux), or plain oatmeal with a dash of salt, cinnamon, and honey or applesauce. For a lighter pre-bed snack, you might also consider tart cherries (or tart cherry juice) or kiwi. I suspect they'll trigger my acid reflux so I've never tried them before bed, but they are both shown to be especially helpful to sleep. (See more on sleep nutrition in the next chapter.)

I'll never know exactly how much this strategy contributed to my sleep improvement, but I do know that my sleep did improve, and once it did, the acid reflux that I'd had for at least seven years virtually disappeared—even though I was still eating only an hour before bedtime.

Now that my schedule has changed, spacing out meals and bedtime is more logistically easy. But I still try to remember to have a light snack roughly two hours before bed. I've found, at least for now, this is my sweet spot. An hour before is okay, but I sometimes get mild reflux. More than two hours before and I'm pretty much guaranteed to wake up hungry.

THE FASTING FIX:
TIME-RESTRICTED EATING

For more on how meal timing can affect circadian rhythm, see chapter 11.

CHAPTER 19

Sleep Nutrition

FOOD AND SLEEP HAVE A bidirectional relationship, meaning they each have an impact on the other. Unfortunately, we know very little about one of those directions.

As a rare expert in both sleep and nutrition, Dr. Marie-Pierre St-Onge says she learned this the hard way in 2015 when the dietary guidelines advisory committee to the U.S. government asked her about guidelines pertaining to sleep. St-Onge, the director of the Sleep Center of Excellence at Columbia University Irving Medical Center, says there was so little reliable information available, her team couldn't make a single recommendation. "We have a lot of information about how sleep influences food intake," she tells me. "But the other side of that, the opposite relationship—diet's influence on sleep—hasn't been studied to that same extent."

This is especially problematic for those with sleep problems, because the science is pretty clear that sleep deprivation leads us to eat more frequently and consume more calories, more saturated fats, and more snacks. So it's commonly advised that people should get more sleep to improve their diet, but if your problem to begin with is difficulty sleeping, that doesn't help at all. What we need is guidance on the other direction: How can we use our diets to improve our sleep?

St-Onge is now on a mission to answer that question. She's conducted a number of comprehensive reviews analyzing existing research and hopes to conduct more extensive studies in the next few years. In the meantime, science can still suggest some nutritional issues that may be contributing to our sleep problems and how to fix them.

Note: The federal government advises that we get most of our nutrients from food. Supplements carry potential side effects and are not regulated in the same way drugs are. For these reasons I'm focusing on food in most of the Fixes below. That said, if you and your doctor decide that supplements are the best way for you to boost your intake, by all means. Sticking to brands that have been verified by third parties like the U.S. Pharmacopeia Convention (USP), NSF International, ConsumerLab.com, or UL, LLC will help ensure that the ingredients on the label accurately represent what's inside. Also, be sure you get the dosing and the timing right to better your chances of sleep improvement.

THE MULTIPURPOSE FIX:
MAGNESIUM

Magnesium is so critical for sleep that it's often referred to as "the sleep mineral." Among its many benefits, research has shown that magnesium helps maintain healthy levels of the neurotransmitter GABA, which, according to the National Sleep Foundation, "is responsible for slowing your thinking down and helping you fall asleep." It's also believed to help reduce cortisol, stress, and anxiety. This can explain why people with low magnesium often experience restless or "broken" sleep. As mentioned earlier, some studies even suggest magnesium can help reduce symptoms of restless legs syndrome and periodic limb movement disorder.

Dan Harris says magnesium has been a big help with what he calls his "ferocious restlessness" at night. "I had been planning to go get a sleep study to get to the bottom of it. I mentioned that to my shrink, who said, 'Why don't you first try magnesium?' Which nobody had ever mentioned to me before. So I started taking it every day, and I would say there's been a well over 50 or 60 or 70 percent reduction in restlessness at bedtime," he tells me.

Recommended Dietary Allowances (RDAs) for Magnesium

Age	Male	Female	Pregnancy	Lactation
Birth to 6 months	30 mg*	30 mg*		
7–12 months	75 mg*	75 mg*		
1–3 years	80 mg	80 mg		
4–8 years	130 mg	130 mg		
9–13 years	240 mg	240 mg		
14–18 years	410 mg	360 mg	400 mg	360 mg
19–30 years	400 mg	310 mg	350 mg	310 mg
31–50 years	420 mg	320 mg	360 mg	320 mg
51+ years	420 mg	320 mg		

Based on chart from the National Institutes of Health

*Adequate Intake (AI)

Despite its importance, it's estimated up to a third of Americans may qualify as magnesium deficient, and roughly half of Americans don't meet their recommended daily allowance (RDA). Even some who do meet their RDA might still be deficient, because magnesium helps the body absorb calcium, phosphorus, and vitamin D. The more of those nutrients you consume, the more magnesium you need.

Unfortunately, testing for magnesium deficiency is difficult because less than 1 percent of the body's magnesium is stored in the blood. Which means a blood test could show normal magnesium levels even in someone with a significant deficiency.

To ensure you're getting enough magnesium, load up on magnesium-rich foods like green leafy vegetables, beans, nuts, seeds, whole grains, magnesium-fortified cereals, and magnesium-rich water.

Supplements are also an option, but in high doses they can cause diarrhea, stomach upset, and in extreme cases magnesium toxicity. They can also interact with other medications, so you'll definitely want to consult your doctor before adding supplements to your diet.

Finally, another increasingly marketed method of upping magnesium intake is through topical magnesium oils, creams, or sprays. So far these have not shown significant efficacy in clinical studies, and I have to say I found these did nothing for me. That said, many of these studies suggest future studies should look at higher dosage of topical magnesium for longer durations, and anecdotally many still swear by it, including my friend and dermatologist Teresa Ishak. "I've just tried a lot of different things for sleep . . . and then I came across something online [about magnesium spray]. I tried it, and the first night I saw it helped my sleep. I haven't had sleep problems since."

It's worth noting the placebo effect on insomnia has been shown to be "remarkably robust and durable." So it's possible that's what Ishak and others who swear by topical magnesium are experiencing. But unlike oral magnesium supplements, Ishak says transdermal magnesium carries little risk of side effects, so it's a low-risk experiment. "It can itch for like a minute, up to five minutes afterward, and that's probably the only rate-limiting factor of people not wanting to use magnesium topically," she says.

Still, as with any other remedy, check with your doctor before trying it.

THE E-ZPASS FIX:
TRYPTOPHAN + CARBS = SEROTONIN

Tryptophan is most talked about around Thanksgiving, since it's found in turkey and is often blamed for the Thanksgiving "food coma." How much of your post-meal sleepiness is due to the turkey is debatable, but it is true that tryptophan is a precursor of both serotonin, which helps regulate mood, and melatonin. A 2016 review also found tryptophan has been shown to increase subjective sleepiness, and sleep quality, while tryptophan deficiency inhibits REM sleep and can lead to depression, anxiety, and other mood disorders, which also impact sleep.

When it comes to tryptophan, the general issue is not that we don't consume enough of it. A 2016 study found most Americans actually get more than their recommended daily intake of tryptophan. But that's only part of the story.

Once ingested, tryptophan still has to make it to the brain and be converted into serotonin to have its desired effect on sleep, and to get there it has to compete with many other amino acids. It's like a bottleneck of traffic, and tryptophan, the least plentiful amino acid, has a particularly tough time getting through.

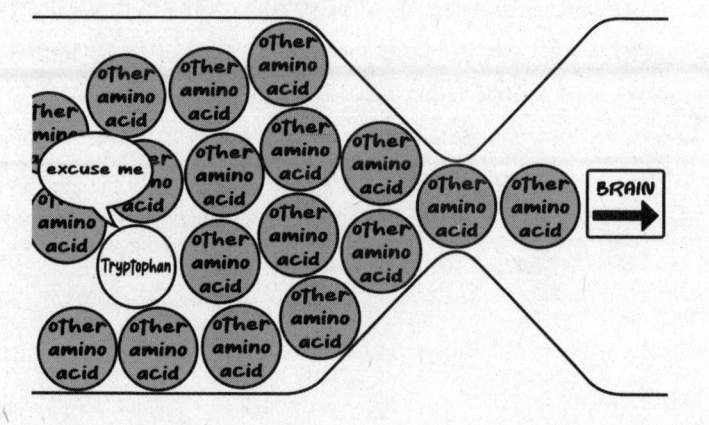

Luckily, carbs are like E-ZPass for tryptophan. The National Sleep Foundation writes: "Carbohydrates cause your body to release insulin, which removes all amino acids—except tryptophan—from your blood. That means that tryptophan has no competition and can enter the brain easily, boosting serotonin levels." So your Thanksgiving food coma likely has as much to do with your giant helping of sweet potatoes and stuffing as it does your giant helping of turkey.

This is especially helpful for chronic insomniacs, who can use that serotonin hit to counter their elevated nighttime cortisol levels. Yet almost every diet currently on trend has one thing in common: a dramatic reduction in carbohydrates.

Current studies on how these diets impact sleep are pretty limited and make it almost impossible to distinguish whether the results are due to a decrease in carbohydrates or an increase in things like fat and protein. But it is common for people to complain of sleep troubles after switching to a low-carb diet, at least at first. So if you have trouble sleeping and adhere to a low-carb diet, it's worth considering whether that might be contributing to your problem.

It's also worth noting that carbs and tryptophan don't have to be consumed at the same time, because carbs can react with tryptophan that's already stored in the body. So while you might think it's better to eat carbs early in the day so you have time to "burn them off," many sleep experts advise those with trouble falling asleep do the opposite. Eat protein-heavy meals earlier, and carbs later in the day, so you can capitalize on that stored tryptophan.

Just be sure to choose complex carbs from whole grains, as opposed to simple carbs like white bread, regular pasta, or anything sugary. These can cause blood sugar spikes, potentially impairing sleep.

THE CONVERSION FIX:
VITAMIN B$_6$

While carbs help tryptophan reach the brain, it still has to be converted into serotonin once it gets there. That's where vitamin B$_6$ comes in. Among its many functions, vitamin B$_6$ plays a crucial role in synthesizing tryptophan into both serotonin and then melatonin. According to the Alaska Sleep Clinic, B$_6$ deficiency is linked to "lowered serotonin levels and poor sleep" as well as "symptoms of depression and mood disorders which can lead to insomnia."

But, while a 2003–2004 survey showed most Americans consume the recommended amounts of vitamin B$_6$, 24 percent of those who didn't take supplements still had low B$_6$ blood levels. Even among people who did take supplements, 11 percent had low levels. So you might want to aim a bit higher than the RDA, being careful not to exceed the upper limits for both food and supplement intakes of vitamin B$_6$.

Recommended Dietary Allowances (RDAs) for Vitamin B6

Age	Male	Female	Pregnancy	Lactation
Birth to 6 months	0.1 mg*	0.1 mg*		
7–12 months	0.3 mg*	0.3 mg*		
1–3 years	0.5 mg	0.5 mg		
4–8 years	0.6 mg	0.6 mg		
9–13 years	1.0 mg	1.0 mg		
14–18 years	1.3 mg	1.2 mg	1.9 mg	2.0 mg
19–50 years	1.3 mg	1.3 mg	1.9 mg	2.0 mg
51+ years	1.7 mg	1.5 mg		

*Adequate Intake (AI)

Based on chart from The National Institutes of Health

Tolerable Upper Intake Levels (ULs) For Vitamin B6

Age	Male / Female
Birth To 6 Months	(Not possible To establish*
7-12 months	(Not possible To establish*
1-3 years	30 mg
4-8 years	40 mg
9-13 years	60 mg
14-18 years	80 mg
19+ years	100 mg

Based on chart From The National Institutes of Health

* Breast milk, Formula, and Food should be The only sources of vitamin B6 For infants.

As for what to eat to raise your vitamin B$_6$ intake, two of the richest sources are fish and organ meats, but according to the National Institutes of Health, most American adults get their dietary B$_6$ from fortified cereals, beef, poultry, starchy vegetables, and non-citrus fruits.

As a bonus, a 2018 study found vitamin B$_6$ can also help us to remember our dreams.

THE EXTRA HELP FIX:
VITAMIN D

Despite its name, vitamin D is actually considered more of a hormone than a vitamin because we can access it without consuming anything. All you have to do is get some sun and your kidneys will produce it. But it's estimated almost 50 percent of the population worldwide doesn't get a sufficient amount of vitamin D. In addition to being problematic for bone health and a number of other issues, that's also problematic for sleep.

Recommended Dietary Allowances (RDAs) For Vitamin D

Age	Male / Female
0–12 months* *Adequate Intake	10 mcg (400 IU)
1–13 years	15 mcg (600 IU)
14–70 years	15 mcg (600 IU)
>70 years	20 mcg (800 IU)

Based on chart from the National Institutes of Health

A 2018 meta-analysis found a significant association between low levels of vitamin D and an increased risk of sleep disorders, including poor sleep quality, short sleep duration, and sleepiness. And while I wondered if this was just an indication of lack of sunlight, which we already know can be detrimental to sleep, the meta-analysis also showed evidence that vitamin D has a positive impact on sleep disorders, even without sunlight. Studies have also linked vitamin D deficiency to obstructive sleep apnea—the lower the vitamin D levels, the more severe the apnea.

Vitamin D from the Sun

It's difficult to know how much sun exposure we would need to meet our vitamin D goals, because factors like geographical location, time of day, cloud cover, skin tone, skin exposure, and sunscreen all impact your vitamin D intake.

But according to the National Institutes of Health, it is currently unknown if there's any way to get vitamin D from the sun without increased risk of skin cancer. So you're probably better off sticking with a broad-spectrum sunscreen and upping your vitamin D intake through other means.

Vitamin D from Food

Ideally we would get all our needed Vitamin D from our diet. The problem is very few foods naturally contain vitamin D—basically just fish, egg yolks, and mushrooms. And even when you factor in fortified foods, very few provide the 10–19% Daily Value needed to be considered "good sources" of vitamin D.

So while the *Dietary Guidelines for America* advise getting most of our nutrients from food, Harvard Medical School says on its website that most people require supplements to get enough vitamin D. That said, Harvard also warns you should still get as much vitamin D from food as possible and not overdo it on supplements, advising "you probably don't need more than 600 to 800 IU per day."

THE FAT FIX:
RIGHT FATS, RIGHT TIME

While carbs are now public enemy number one in the weight-loss world, fat is largely out of the doghouse. In fact, many weight-loss diets now promote a high intake of fat. But this can be problematic for sleep, especially for those struggling with waking throughout the night.

In a 2016 study, Dr. St-Onge and other researchers found higher fat intakes, particularly saturated fat, were associated with less deep sleep. Unfortunately, St-Onge says we still don't know why this is— one of the many areas of sleep nutrition that needs further research.

What we do know is, Americans generally consume too much saturated fat. Only 29 percent of us get less than 10 percent of our calories from saturated fat as recommended by the dietary guidelines. And the American Heart Association says we really should be shooting for under 6 percent. With the right strategy this might be easier than you think.

How-To: Cut Down on Saturated Fats

For me, the easiest way to cut down on saturated fats, which are solid at room temperature, was to swap them with unsaturated fats, which are liquid at room temperature. Saturated fats often come from meat and dairy, while unsaturated fats generally come from vegetables, nuts, seeds, and fish. Think olive oil instead of butter.

The Dietary Guidelines for Americans also suggest:

- choosing lean cuts of meat, grilled instead of fried
- replacing some meat in tacos, stir-fries, or other mixed dishes, with fish, beans, or other vegetables
- limiting desserts to special occasions and choosing fresh fruit when possible
- using smaller plates and bowls to encourage smaller portions

Finally, a tip inspired by Chef Rocco DiSpirito: If you like deep-fried food, try flash frying instead. To do this precook the food first by braising or microwaving, then fry at 400 degrees just long enough to brown the outside. This can be as short as 10 seconds. The food absorbs a fraction of the oil, but still has that nice deep-fried crunch. If you have an air fryer, that's also a great alternative.

Timing

Despite all the tips above, every now and then only butter will do. So if you still want to indulge in saturated fat, you might want to consider *when* you eat it. A 2016 study that looked at nutritional data for nearly 1,500 Chinese adults over five years found that "the association between fat intake and sleep varies according to how late or how early in the day a meal is eaten." While high-fat dinners were associated with persistent short sleep, high-fat breakfasts were actually helpful in preventing daytime sleepiness.

The study didn't differentiate between types of fat, but it still seems reasonable to deduce that if you're going to indulge in something with saturated fats, you're better off enjoying it earlier in the day, rather than in the evening.

THE LIGHT SLEEP FIX:
FIBER

Fiber is probably best known for its ability to relieve constipation and keep us "regular," but fiber has many other benefits too—including helping us stay asleep. In the 2016 study cited above, Dr. St-Onge and her team found low fiber intake—like high fat intake—was associated with lighter, less restorative sleep.

Yet low fiber is the norm for most of us. According to the USDA, we should take in 14 grams of fiber for every 1,000 calories we consume. Americans on average get only about half of that.

Reasons for this include the popularity of ultra-processed foods, refined or simple carbs, and low-carb and gluten-free diets. Also, while whole grains are naturally high in fiber, many products labeled "whole grain" still don't meet the FDA's definition of a good source of fiber. That means even those of us trying to eat healthy are probably getting a lot less fiber than we think. Instead, when buying packaged food, check the label. If the product has at least 2.5 grams of fiber per serving, it's considered a good source of fiber. If it contains 5 or more grams of fiber per serving, it's considered an excellent source of fiber.

Other foods high in fiber include legumes, beans, vegetables, fruits, nuts, and seeds.

Finally, it's important to note, upping your fiber intake should be a gradual process. Adding too much too quickly can lead to gas, bloating, and cramping. The Mayo Clinic recommends reaching your fiber goal "over a few weeks" and to stay hydrated, as "fiber works best when it absorbs water."

THE MIDNIGHT PEE FIX:
SEE YA, SODIUM

If your sleep problems are due to overnight bathroom trips, you might want to look at your sodium intake. The *Dietary Guidelines for Americans* recommend limiting sodium to 2,300 milligrams per day—basically equivalent to one teaspoon of salt. But Americans average more than 3,400 milligrams a day. The result is an increased risk of medical conditions like high blood pressure, heart disease, and stroke, but also an increased risk of sleep interruptions.

A 2017 study shows that excessive salt intake is an independent risk factor for nighttime urination, aka nocturia, and that this is impacted not only by salt consumed in the evening but also by daytime eating habits. This is especially important among older adults, who often struggle with frequent nighttime urination.

But according to the *Dietary Guidelines for Americans,* more than 70 percent of our sodium intake comes from processed food and restaurant meals—not from our saltshaker. And it doesn't take much to surpass the recommended limit. The CDC says a bowl of cereal with skim milk for breakfast, a cup of soup and a turkey sandwich for lunch, and a slice of pizza with a lightly dressed salad for dinner can put you well over the top. Still, some simple adjustments can go a long way.

How-To: Cut Down on Sodium

Here are some tips from the CDC, the Mayo Clinic, and the FDA:

- When eating frozen or canned foods, choose low-sodium versions, and avoid options that come in a sauce.
- Rinse canned foods to remove some of the sodium.

(continued on next page)

- Read nutrition labels. Seek out lower sodium versions of your favorite foods and try to avoid anything with more than 200 milligrams of sodium per serving. (More on decoding label info below.)
- Avoid processed meat and poultry "enhanced" with salt water or saline.
- If using sauces or prepackaged seasonings, opt for low-sodium options and/or use small amounts rather than the whole packet.
- Remove salt from recipes or add salt only after tasting.
- If eating out, ask that salt not be added to your meal, request sauces and dressings on the side, and/or ask for low-sodium options.
- Don't overdo it with salt substitutes. You can still get too much sodium and risk getting too much potassium as well.

It's also worth knowing what sodium claims actually mean. Here they are in order of preference:

- "Sodium Free" = less than 5 milligrams of sodium per serving
- "Very Low Sodium" = 35 milligrams of sodium or less per serving
- "Low Sodium" = 140 milligrams of sodium or less per serving
- "Lite" or "Light" in Sodium = at least 50 percent less sodium than the regular version (but may still be high in sodium)
- "Reduced Sodium" = at least 25 percent less sodium than the regular version (but may still be high in sodium)
- "No Salt Added" or "Unsalted" = no salt added, but may still include ingredients high in sodium. This is not that same as "Sodium Free."

If you find reducing sodium challenging, take comfort in knowing your taste buds will adjust. Just move gradually toward your goal. Not only will you start to miss salt less, you may even start preferring less salt.

THE COMPREHENSIVE FIX:
MEDITERRANEAN DIET

There is currently no scientifically backed "sleep diet" per se, but there is a growing body of literature supporting the positive impacts of the Mediterranean diet on sleep. In a 2019 review, St-Onge describes several epidemiological studies that found greater adherence to Mediterranean diet correlated with lower likelihood of insomnia and lower likelihood of poor sleep quality.

And while she says clinical trials are needed to determine if it is the diet that's causing the good sleep, there are a few explanations for why it could, including that the Mediterranean diet:

- is high in fiber
- is high in magnesium
- is high in tryptophan
- is high in complex carbs
- is low in saturated fat
- has a beneficial effect on gut microbiome
- promotes weight loss for those who are overweight, which can also positively impact sleep

How-To: Mediterranean Diet

There's no single definition for the Mediterranean diet, but it's generally high in fruits, vegetables, whole grains, nuts, seeds, and olive oil, with moderate amounts of fish and poultry and very limited red meat.

For a smooth transition, the Harvard Health blog recommends implementing one change a week from the list below, starting with whatever you think will be easiest:

- *Olive Oil:* Gradually swap out other fats for extra-virgin olive oil in hot dishes, salads, or even on bread.
- *Nuts and Olives:* Replace processed snacks with a handful of raw nuts or olives.
- *Whole Grains:* Stick to whole grain options for carbs like bread, pasta, and rice, and try other whole grains like bulgur, barley, farro, and couscous.
- *Salad:* Start or end each meal with a salad of crisp dark greens and vegetables.
- *Vegetables:* Add extra veggies to meals, aiming for four servings a day.
- *Legumes:* Eat at least three servings of legumes like lentils, chickpeas, beans, and peas per week.
- *Less Meat:* Eat lean poultry in 3- to 4-ounce portions and eat lean red meat only occasionally. Make sure meat is accompanied by a lot of vegetables.
- *Fish:* Aim for two to three servings of canned or fresh fish a week.
- *Wine:* Replace other alcoholic beverages with wine, "but no more than two 5-ounce glasses per day for men and one glass per day for women."
- *Beverages:* Drink water in place of juice or soda.
- *Fruit:* "Aim for three servings of fresh fruit a day."
- *Dessert:* Save fatty sugary desserts for special occasions and stick to healthy options like poached or fresh fruit for every day.

THE LIQUID FIX:
SLEEP-FRIENDLY BEVERAGES

When it comes to helping sleep, beverages often get more attention than food. Some swear by a glass of warm milk, others by their favorite herbal tea. But St-Onge says the only sleep-improving beverage with solid scientific backing is one you may never even have heard of: tart cherry juice. She adds that teas like valerian tea or chamomile tea "may have a calming effect."

Just remember to think of these foods and beverages as something that might *enhance* your sleep, not something that's going to *make* you sleep. As Dr. Chris Winter writes in his book *The Sleep Solution*, "If you are getting to a place where you feel you can no longer sleep without your cup of chamomile tea and bowl full of dried tart cherries, it's time to back up and put these foods in their proper place . . . an option, not a necessity."

THE ANNOYING FIX:
FOOD DIARY APP

If you've read the previous chapters, you know by now that food is not something I sacrifice easily. But the worse my insomnia got, the worse my eating habits got. At the time I didn't know all the science that I do now, but even then I knew I had to do something.

Perfectly tracking my every calorie is not generally my thing. But for a short period of time, I did keep a food diary via the My-FitnessPal app, and I found it surprisingly helpful. By automatically calculating the nutritional info for most food, the app gave me a much clearer picture of what I was ingesting every day and where my problems areas were. It also helped me be more thoughtful about my eating habits and opened my eyes to how much mindless snacking I was doing—mainly as a source of comfort for my sleep problems.

This doesn't mean I never indulged in unhealthy food. But it made me think twice about it, because I knew I couldn't just shove a handful of fries in my mouth and forget about it minutes later. I would have to write that down and directly see the impact it had on my nutritional count for the day—which annoyed my competitive side. Instead, I'd consider indulgences and ask myself, *Do I really want this? Is it worth it?* Sometimes the answer would be no, and I would skip it. Sometimes the answer would be yes, and I would make it a point to thoroughly enjoy those fries—with no regrets.

If I were doing it again today, I would pay more attention to the nutrients mentioned in the Fixes above. I'd also use the app in conjunction with a sleep diary to look for any patterns between my eating habits and my sleep quality—but only if I felt I could do that without getting too obsessive about it. It's not a perfect science, as most of us will have several factors affecting our sleep, and the app itself isn't perfectly accurate. But it might help to connect the dots on whether you, for example, take more overnight bathroom breaks after consuming more sodium, or fall asleep more easily after a carb-centric dinner.

That said, if tracking your diet makes you think and worry more about sleep, stop doing it. The repercussions of increased sleep anxiety will far outweigh any benefits you get from fine-tuning your food intake.

CHAPTER 20

Relaxation Tools

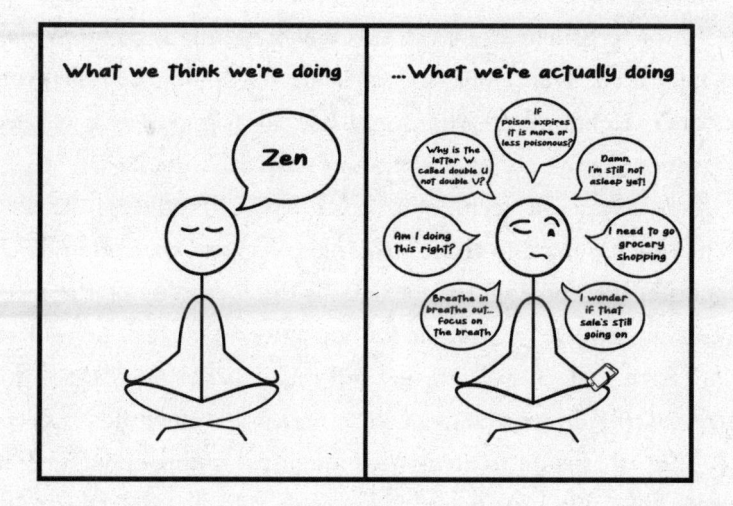

RELAXATION TOOLS ARE OFTEN PEDDLED as a magic formula for sleep. One article promises "4–7–8 breathing" will help you "fall asleep in 60 seconds or less." A YouTube video "guarantees" the so-called military method will get you to sleep "in as little as 10 seconds." And a guest backstage at GMA once assured me, "Breathe in through your right nostril, then out through your left nostril—you'll pass out, I promise."

Spoiler alert: none of these worked for me. And if you've read chapter 3, you already know how trying to meditate myself to sleep worked out. All of it left me feeling hopeless and broken. Several sleep specialists tell me this is not a unique experience.

But I have some good news for others feeling this way. The problem isn't that we're broken or that these methods are useless. The problem is: The idea that anything will get us to sleep in seconds or minutes, is, in the words of Dr. Michael Grandner, "bullshit."

For starters, healthy adults generally take roughly ten to twenty minutes to fall asleep. If you fall asleep much faster than this, it's not a good thing—it's an indication that you are sleep-deprived and potentially have a sleep disorder.

Second, even if you ignore their ridiculous time claims, these false promises perpetuate the myth that any one thing is going to *make* us fall asleep. That alone can set us up for failure. Because while it's easier to fall asleep when we're relaxed as opposed to aroused, relaxation doesn't *put* us to sleep, our sleep drive does.

Also, relaxation techniques don't always produce relaxation. When we use them to try to make sleep happen, they often do the opposite. We don't appreciate the breathing exercise or the meditation or any other technique for how it makes us feel. Instead, we work hard to do it well, so that it'll make us sleep. All that effort makes our brain more active, which makes it even harder to sleep.

"When I attempt to meditate, I am just thinking about whether or not I'm doing a good job meditating," my colleague Trevor Ault tells me. "I can't think beyond, 'Okay, and now I'm meditating . . . I'm meditating. . . . All, right I think that this is meditating, is it working?'"

Whit Johnson says he once tried using a special light that shines onto the ceiling and swells and compresses to guide users into an ideal breathing rhythm for sleep. "I found that to be absolute torture!" he tells me. "I cannot breathe on that rhythm to save my life." Whit's inability to stay on that breathing rhythm would then make him so anxious that he felt like he couldn't breathe at all. "I would start having panic attacks!" he says.

Dr. Jason Ong, who specializes in mindfulness and insomnia, says it's the fact that we want to sleep so badly that causes our stress. "So anything you do to try to make sleep happen is likely going to backfire," he tells me. "Whether it's meditation, whether it's deep breathing, it doesn't really matter what it is—the harder you try to sleep, the less likely you're going to sleep."

As explained in chapter 3, it's like we're trying to sleep and also continuously asking ourselves, *Are you asleep yet?!* The obvious answer is *No, because you won't SHUT UP!* What we really need to do is chill out and stop putting so much pressure on ourselves to fall asleep so we can drift off when our body is ready to. Relaxation techniques can help with that—if we have the right attitude and understanding.

That said, relaxation techniques are unlikely to be effective on their own against established insomnia. So rather than get frustrated that relaxation techniques aren't "working" for you, read chapter 3 of this book to see if you have conditioned arousal. If so, start with the tools in part 2 first. Then use the tools in this chapter as a way to further your progress.

It's also worth noting that relaxation techniques can affect people differently. If any of these techniques make you feel more energized, that may be a cue that they'll make a better addition to your daytime routine than to your nighttime routine, which can still be beneficial for sleeping. And if a technique makes you feel more anxious or unstable in any way, stop doing it entirely and contact a mental health professional about what you're experiencing.

THE FOUNDATIONAL FIX:
DO CONSTRUCTIVE WORRY FIRST

If you haven't already read chapter 3, please do—or at the very least, read the section on constructive worry. There's a reason that tool is singled out in the beginning of this book and isn't just another relaxation method quickly mentioned in this chapter. Virtually every behavioral sleep specialist I've asked agrees that constructive worry, sometimes referred to as scheduled worry or worry time, is in a category all its own when it comes to lowering the arousal that disrupts our sleep.

Constructive worry also helped to put me in a state of mind that allowed me to use other relaxation tools successfully, which is why I highly recommend starting with constructive worry so you can lay the foundation for all the other methods mentioned in this chapter.

THE INTENTION FIX:
DO THE EXERCISE FOR ITS OWN SAKE

To keep relaxation or mental exercises from backfiring, the first thing we have to do is stop viewing them as a sleep tool and start viewing them as something to enjoy for their own sake. As Dr. Daniel Erichsen explains, "If you have any type of relaxation technique, and you look at that as simply a way to feel good, feel relaxed, enjoy, and you think of it as, 'This thing I'm doing is a gift in itself, it is not a means to an end,' then it can be helpful, because it takes attention away from sleep."

Erichsen says this even holds true with passive activities like watching TV. He says if you watch TV with the intention of escaping anxious thoughts, "That's the problem, because you're trying to escape those thoughts, you bottle them up inside you, and then as soon as you turn off the TV, they all come back at you . . . but when the intent is simply, 'Hey, I want to watch this show because I like it'—no problem at all."

By appreciating the exercise rather than focusing on whether it'll make us sleep, we shift the voice in our head away from constantly asking if we're asleep yet and instead direct its attention to thoughts like *Mmmm, I like how this makes me feel.*

THE MINDSET FIX:
HAVE A PASSIVE ATTITUDE

As I explained in chapter 3, my first few attempts at meditation did not go well, mostly because I couldn't keep myself from getting distracted. That made me really frustrated—which made me more awake.

I didn't know at the time that my wandering mind wasn't the problem. The problem was my *attitude* toward my wandering mind. I finally learned this when I listened to a mindfulness meditation by my colleague Dan Harris for the first time. In true Dan form, the meditation was called "Proof That You Don't Suck at Meditation." I hit play, and there was Dan telling me to focus on the breath, but with the same casual tone in his voice as when he tells me to not embarrass him a second before we're about to go live on air, or when he compliments all my hard work—after a segment in which I haven't said anything. Hearing my mischievous friend guiding a meditation was funny at first, but then I had an aha moment when he said in the recording, "Sooner or later . . . your mind is going to go nuts. As soon as you notice you've become distracted, that's a win!" This moment that I'd continuously viewed as a failure, Dan says is actually "the moment of success."

"That's the whole point of meditation is to notice distraction, over and over and over again," he tells me. He calls this a "bicep curl for your brain," which over time helps with attention regulation and, as Dan puts it, "allows you not to be so yanked around or owned or governed by all of your emotions and neurotic obsessions."

For me, just knowing that mind wandering is both normal and expected made a huge difference. I was finally able to stop getting upset about my wandering mind and just accept it. This is something sleep experts call a passive attitude, which they largely consider to be the most important ingredient in achieving relaxation.

THE TRAINING WHEELS FIX:
PRACTICE

You wouldn't play the piano for the first time blindfolded at a concert, but so many of us try relaxation exercises for the first time when we're really anxious and when we're desperate for sleep—so we're starting from a disadvantage *and* the stakes are high.

Instead, sleep specialists generally recommend practicing relaxation daily when you're not particularly stressed. This way you can develop the skill *before* you try doing it when you're more anxious. If you do the exercise enough times while you're relaxed, your brain also starts to associate the exercise with relaxation, and then the exercise becomes a cue for relaxation. Eventually just starting up your meditation app, for example, can trigger the brain to think *Oh, I know what this means—it's time to relax.* This classical conditioning makes whatever technique you're using that much more effective when you need it most.

THE FLEXIBLE FIX:
EXPERIMENT

Progressive muscle relaxation, autogenic training, mindfulness meditation, and imagery are the relaxation techniques that get the most attention related to sleep. Good information and guides on those are easy to find, so I won't bother breaking down each one in detail. But, as explained in the *BSM Treatment Protocols for Sleep Disorders* textbook, "The possible modifications and variants of relaxation are likely infinite," so experiment to see what works best for you.

Dr. Michael Grandner tells me his rule of thumb is: "If someone is stuck in their head, get them into their body. And if someone is stuck in their body, get them into their head." If you feel aroused because of physical pain or discomfort, Grandner says to try a mental exercise like guided imagery or mindfulness meditation. If you feel like you're stuck in your head, try something more physical like progressive muscle relaxation, stretches, or breath work.

Breath work instructor Eliza Kane, who, full disclosure, is also a personal friend of mine, suggests the following technique:

How-To: Breath Work Meditation

1. Find a time where you can lie down for 15 to 20 minutes with no distractions. At first, choose a time when you're already fairly relaxed.
2. Lie on your back and put one hand on your lower abdomen and the other on your chest.
3. Through your mouth, inhale half a breath into your abdomen, then inhale the other half into your upper chest, and then exhale. You should be able to feel each respective hand rise as you do the two-part inhale. These do not have to be big breaths, just whatever feels comfortable. Again, this is all through the mouth, not the nose.
4. Find a rhythm that feels good to you and repeat step 3 for 15 to 20 minutes.

(continued on next page)

5. You can opt to listen to music as you do this. This can help you to naturally fall into a rhythm and can make it even more enjoyable. Eliza suggests something more upbeat but relaxing to start, and then something slower and more soothing toward the end.
6. If at any point you notice you got distracted, that's totally fine. Just find your rhythm again and carry on.
7. It's normal to feel sensations like tingling or vibrations, but if you find the exercise is making you feel more anxious in any way, do not continue.

You'll notice I stressed twice that this technique is to be done through the open mouth. That's important, not only because of the effect of the breath itself but also because breathing through our nose is automatic. Eliza says since breathing through our mouth does not come naturally, our brain has to pay attention just to do the exercise, which helps shift our attention away from our anxieties and racing thoughts. To me, it felt like meditation with training wheels, where I didn't have to try so hard to focus on the breath because the exercise itself generates that focus.

"It's an active meditation . . . it satiates that part of the mind that feels like it always needs to be doing something," Eliza tells me. In this way, she says, it meets people where they are and "guides them into the relaxation, in a simple and easy way, where they don't have to overthink it."

But Eliza warns there are other more "aggressive" forms of breath work done through the open mouth, like holotropic breath work, that she says can be too intense. "For some people they work really well. For other people, it actually can be really traumatic," she explains.

So Eliza recommends sticking to this more "gentle" technique. If you want guided options that use it, you can find them on her website, ElizaRoseKane.com. She also recommends David Elliott Meditations on Spotify, which are free.

As always, if something feels off at any point—during any kind of meditation—stop and contact a professional.

Finally, it's also important to note your experimentation with relaxation can go beyond traditional techniques. Dr. Daniel Erichsen suggests just doing something you enjoy, whatever that thing is. "Some people like audiobooks, play some piano, do something that is a gift in itself," he says, but most importantly, "make bedtime something to look forward to."

CHAPTER 21

Rethinking the Bedtime Routine

IF YOU'VE DONE ANY READING on sleep, you've probably heard about the importance of a bedtime routine, and for good reason: a good bedtime routine can be very beneficial—but those of us with sleep problems don't always reap the benefits.

That's because one of the main benefits of a bedtime routine is its classical conditioning effect. You might remember from chapter 3, this is when the brain recognizes familiar patterns and starts to anticipate what's coming next. So if you have a set of rituals that consistently end in sleep—for example, watching TV, having some tea, brushing your teeth, reading a book—your brain will start to recognize those rituals as a cue to prepare for sleep. This is why we often have bedtime routines for kids, like bath time and story time. These rituals are aimed at helping kids wind down at night, but if you do them consistently, they also send a signal to the child's brain that bath time means it's time to prepare for sleep, and story time means they're even closer to sleep. And the brain powers down a little bit more each step of the way. As Dr. Michael Grandner puts it, "The brain is a pattern recognition machine. Feed it a pattern—a routine that brings you to sleep—and it will recognize it" and help prepare you for sleep "even if other areas of life are erratic."

The problem is, this only works if your bedtime routine consistently ends in sleep. As explained in chapter 3, if your bedtime routine consistently ends with you stressed out and awake in bed, the bedtime routine will instead become a cue for that. And your brain revs up during your bedtime routine, instead of winding down.

Even the more immediate winding-down effect of a bedtime routine works only if we find the rituals themselves relaxing—but insomniacs often don't. We typically fill our bedtime routines with things we feel we *should* do in order to sleep, rather than things we *want* to do because that's how we like to end our day. Plus, when we are doing things we normally find relaxing, our intention often changes. We're no longer sitting in our warm bath enjoying how the water feels against our skin, we're sitting there hoping this bath will help us sleep tonight and worrying about what will happen if it doesn't. This doesn't help our sleep; if anything, it makes things worse. The same can happen if we cut out activities that do relax us, like watching TV.

So instead of changing things in your bedtime routine to try to fix your sleep problems, first ask yourself if a change in your bedtime routine *caused* your sleep problems. If you notice that you started having trouble sleeping when you started playing Grand Theft Auto in the evening, or checking emails before bed, or having an extra glass of wine at dinner, then change those things and see if that fixes the problem. If the *timing* of your bedtime routine has changed, due to a new work schedule for example, your sleep problems might also be related to your circadian rhythm. Check out part 3 of this book for more on that.

If not, and if you don't suspect any of the other conditions described in chapter 1, chances are the real problem is that your bed and bedtime routine have become a cue for wakefulness instead of sleep, aka conditioned arousal. No amount of Sleepytime tea or bubble baths is going to fix that. Instead, try the evidence-based techniques in part 2 of this book. Then use the Fixes below to help reinforce those techniques with a bedtime routine you can look forward to.

THE FLASHBACK FIX:
BEDTIME BACKTRACK

When trying to get your bedtime routine back on track, consider starting with a simple question: "What did you do before you had sleep problems?"

Dr. Jennifer Mundt, a sleep psychologist and assistant professor at Northwestern Feinberg School of Medicine, says her patients will typically come in saying, "I stopped using screens, and I went to blue-blocking glasses, and I'm reading and doing everything, and I still can't sleep." But when asked what they used to do when they slept fine, she says they typically respond: "I just watched TV and went to bed. I didn't think about it." She says if you used to sleep fine after watching TV, the TV and the blue light weren't the problem. "People are changing things that actually don't need to be changed."

All these changes then make us obsess more about sleep, because we're working so hard to make sleep happen. Unfortunately, as explained in chapter 3, in doing that we put a lot of pressure on ourselves to fall asleep, which raises our arousal, gives us performance anxiety, and ultimately keeps us awake.

So if you can, go back to whatever you used to do before sleep became a problem . . . back before you even realized you had a bedtime routine.

THE CUSTOMIZED FIX:
THERE IS NO FORMULA

If you never liked your bedtime routine, it can be tempting to spend hours, days, or even weeks researching the "perfect" bedtime routine.

Let me save you a lot of time: there's no such thing. As Dr. Mundt explains, "What is calming for one person is really stimulating for another person, so it really comes down to that individual."

Evening exercise, for example, makes it hard for some people to sleep, while making it easier for others. My husband likes to sleep on an empty stomach; I sleep much better after a light snack.

Even if bedtime routines were universal, as Dr. Jade Wu explains, having a perfect one isn't a good thing—it's a red flag for insomnia. "When people come in and in the first session they tell me they have impeccable sleep hygiene or they have a perfect bedtime routine, I know that there's trouble ahead," she says. That's because having a "perfect" bedtime routine indicates you're thinking a lot about your sleep and working really hard to make it happen: two things that make insomnia worse, not better.

Instead of trying to find a perfect formula, Wu says, just ask yourself, off the top of your head: "What do you think would be nice to do in the roughly hour or half hour before bed?" Then do that. From that point, she says, we should stop thinking about our bedtime routine "unless something specifically causes problems—and it never does."

THE FLEXIBLE FIX:
ROUTINE, NOT RIGID

Just because you like reading at night doesn't mean you have to read every night. Same goes for any part of your bedtime routine. You can even skip the routine entirely—because it's never our bedtime routine that makes us sleep. I like to think of this like the sleep equivalent of a good food commercial. Seeing the food sizzling on the screen might make my mouth water and stoke my appetite, but I don't need to see a food commercial in order to be able to eat.

Our routine also doesn't have to be exactly the same or happen every single night for its conditioning effect to kick in. So instead of trying to mimic a good sleeper's nighttime rituals, mimic their attitude toward those rituals. My husband never misses something enjoyable because he needs to start his bedtime routine—and now neither do I.

THE REMINDER FIX:
THE LAST-CALL ALARM

Sleep experts seem to agree that we all benefit from a period of winding down before bed, but this is less helpful if you go back to frantically crossing off to-do list items after that downtime.

I used to be terrible at this. I would enjoy a relaxing evening of watching TV with my husband, and maybe take a hot bath. But then bedtime would hit, and only then would I realize I still had to send an email, put in a grocery order, and do some other time-sensitive task. Then I'd either stay up late to get those things done or go to bed worrying about them—and take forever to fall asleep. Either way, not ideal.

To help with this, Dr. Michael Grandner suggests setting what I like to call the last-call alarm. Just like a bar informs customers when it's their last chance to get a drink, the last-call alarm is a gentle notice to try to finish whatever tasks you want to get done today or officially put them off until tomorrow.

With your tasks done or officially moved to tomorrow's to-do list, you can be that much more relaxed as you enjoy the rest of the night and finally head to bed.

If you do end up remembering a last-minute thing that needs to get done, that's fine, just do it. No need to freak out. Like almost anything else in this chapter, this strategy is just a bonus to help end your day on a nice note—not a hard-and-fast rule to help you sleep. And as is true with everything else in this book, if you think it'll be helpful, apply it in the way that suits your life best.

I, for example, come home from work, and immediately try to cross off as many to-do list items as I can while my son finishes his nap. When he wakes up, we often squeeze in a quick family trip to the park, and then I make a quick dinner. We eat and have some family time—including our pet rabbit, Frank. Then my son goes to sleep, and my husband and I (and Frank) enjoy some cuddling and TV time together, often just a quick thirty-minute show. When our show is over, that's my last call to myself to finish up any quick, pressing tasks before retreating to our desk in the bedroom to prep for work the next day. When my husband comes in to go to sleep, I turn off the computer, kiss him good night, have a light snack, lay out my clothes for the next day, wash my face, brush my teeth, and sneak into bed. If I'm reporting on a demanding story, get a last-minute assignment, or my work schedule changes—any and all of that routine can go right out the window.

I don't think any sleep article would hail this as a great evening routine, and you'll notice I break many typical sleep rules: my relaxing TV time comes before my work time, I'm on a computer shortly before bed (with f.lux and low brightness), and my workspace is in my bedroom. But we all have to live within the confines of real life. For me, that includes an apartment with limited space, an erratic work schedule for a job that I love, and a family that I want to spend quality time with.

In addition to that, as an anchor for ABC News Live, I cover all the day's top stories, which means I need to be as updated as possible when I go into work in the morning. Since the news cycle changes so quickly, this means I have two choices: read the latest updates at night before bed and then quickly catch up on overnight developments in the morning or wake up even earlier than I already do to get *all* my reading done in the morning. As a night owl, I choose option one because I know that, for me, the benefits of going to sleep and waking up closer to my natural rhythms will far outweigh the negative impacts of my late-night screen time. For my family and me, this is what works best right now. Do what works best for you.

THE SIMPLE FIX:
DON'T OVERTHINK IT

When I started writing this chapter, I thought of my bedtime routine as the period of time between dinner and when I stop working for the night—my family time, my TV time, and my reading/writing time. But after writing it all down, I realize that's arguably not where my bedtime routine ends . . . it's where it begins.

It's the little things that I do after that point, from kissing my husband to washing my face to brushing my teeth: this is my bedtime routine. It just goes to show, your bedtime routine does not need to be long or elaborate. And that snack that I have, I'm only now realizing that I prepare and have it in silence, which unknowingly gives me the chance to process my day—aka unwind.

And *unknowingly* is the key. For all the sleep articles and books that address bedtime routines, most, if not all, miss a key component: for someone predisposed to insomnia, the best thing a bedtime routine can be is effortless, an afterthought.

More importantly, despite all those rules I break, when I lie down in bed at night, I fall asleep, no problem. That was not the case when I had a nearly impeccable bedtime routine . . . but a much less healthy relationship with sleep.

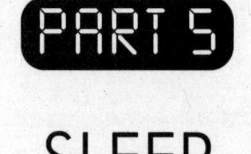

SLEEP
ENVIRONMENT

I know what you're thinking: you can skip this part of the book because you're already familiar with the list of ideal bedroom qualities—keep it cool, dark, quiet, etc. But this isn't just more of the same.

My issue as a struggling insomniac wasn't a lack of material on the general qualities of an ideal bedroom. Instead, it was the lack of detail about how to achieve those ideals, and perhaps more importantly, what to do when the ideal isn't possible. In my case, I tried about twenty different sleep masks, I had earplugs, the AC was cranking, I had lavender oil on my pillow . . . and still I was wide awake.

Of course as a chronic insomniac with a circadian rhythm disorder, I wasn't going to find real relief without addressing the underlying issues that were keeping me awake through the methods explained in parts 2 and 3 of this book. Even the best bedroom setup can't fix that.

But along the way I did learn a bit more about how, despite my best efforts, my sleep environment was working against me.

CHAPTER 22

Let There Be Dark

ONE OF THE BIGGEST ISSUES I had with my sleep environment was too much light in my bedroom. This was extra challenging when I slept during the day, but even before I worked overnights, the room always seemed too light to me. The thing is, I had blackout curtains just like every sleep article suggested, and my husband had no problem falling asleep in that very same room. Eventually I figured the room must be fine, so I must be the problem. It turns out that it was actually a little of both.

Crappy-Eyelid Club

Since long before I was nocturnal, something as subtle as the light from an alarm clock could make it hard for me to sleep. Even now, if my cable box randomly turns on in the middle of the night, that light is enough to wake me. In the process of working on this book, I told a sleep specialist about this and explained that my mother is the exact same way. He basically told me we're waking up for other reasons and just *think* it's the light. But even he admitted he's also heard the same from some of his patients. Is it all in our heads?

Unsatisfied with his answer, I reached out to Dr. Mariana Figueiro, a top expert in the field of how light impacts sleep. She says that while this kind of light sensitivity has yet to be properly studied, it could be due in part to, of all things, our eyelids. "Some people have a lot more [light] transmission through the closed eyelids than others," she tells me. Combine thin eyelids, light-sensitivity, and light sleep, and Figueiro says you could very well have a recipe for someone whose sleep is disturbed with minimal light. So while my room may have been dark enough for my husband—it was not dark enough for me . . . and my crappy eyelids.

The hyperarousal insomniacs often experience at bedtime can also cause pupils to dilate, making our eyes more light sensitive. So for some, you may become less light sensitive as your insomnia improves.

On the off chance this kind of light sensitivity *is* all in our heads, what's in our heads is super important to our sleep, as established in part 2 of this book. So even if making the room darker does nothing but eliminate our worries about too much light, that's still worth it in my book.

Blackout Shmackout

While many articles tout the benefits of a light-tight bedroom, few actually tell you how to get there. I've seen suggestions as vague as "hang window treatments," or my personal favorite: "close the bedroom door." Brilliant! Thanks!

Some get a bit more specific, suggesting blackout curtains. But run a quick internet search for "blackout curtain fail" and you'll quickly see they aren't as foolproof as they sound. For starters, blackout curtains aren't always made of 100 percent light-blocking material. They also generally leave gaps down the center of the curtains and around the perimeter. If you live in a brightly lit city or sleep during the day, this is not going to cut it.

When I was troubleshooting this, I splurged on fancy automatic rolling shades out of desperation. I had asked the saleswoman how effective they were at darkening the room. She replied, "You won't even know there's a window there." I couldn't wait to get them installed!

But when I arrived home to sleep the next morning, my room was not the cave I expected. The shade material, which seemed 100 percent light-blocking, wasn't when hit with direct sunlight. And while I paid extra for light-blocking channels along the sides of the shade, there was a slight gap at the top and bottom. Those gaps let in enough sunlight to illuminate the whole room and, more importantly, disturb my sleep.

Eva Pilgrim had a similar experience when she first installed blackout curtains in her bedroom only to find several gaps letting in light. "You pull the curtains together in the middle . . . then you're pulling the curtains on the end. And then you can't get the light to go away, and then you're annoyed and all worked up about it," she says.

Given all this, I get frustrated when books and articles suggest making the room dark and then move on, as if it's the easiest thing ever. In my experience, creating a "light tight" room is like playing a game of whack-a-mole: as soon as you eliminate one light source, you suddenly notice a new one.

Sleep Masks

By now you might be thinking, "Why doesn't she just wear a sleep mask?"

Sleep masks and earplugs are two of the most commonly recommended sleep tools. And rightfully so: They're cheap, portable, easy to find, and can be a total game changer.

But if you're a light sleeper, as many insomniacs are, the feeling of the sleep mask on your face can disturb your sleep. This may be due at least in part to the fact that the arousal that makes it hard for us to sleep also heightens our senses—including our sense of touch. I tried every type of sleep mask I could find, but I felt like the princess and the pea: one crushed my eyelashes, the next pinched my nose, another one hurt my head, the next let in too much light. Even after I finally found a concave mask that doesn't touch my eyes or lashes and is fully light-blocking, I still tossed and turned, my hair had a weird crease in it, and I ended up taking the thing off long before my wake-up time.

I had a similar experience with earplugs.

Then, more recently, I accidentally discovered that if I stick a nasal strip on the part of the mask that covers my nose, it alleviates the tiny amount of pressure there that I didn't even realize was bothering me. With that adjustment, I can now wear that concave mask with few disruptions to my sleep. This is a game changer when I have to sleep somewhere that isn't completely dark. In a pinch, I've also covered my eyes with a soft T-shirt.

That said, I still don't want to sleep with a mask every night if I don't have to. So by all means try different sleep masks, and if you find one you can sleep through the night in, stop drilling—you've hit oil! But if you find wearing a mask interferes with your sleep, consider the solutions below instead.

THE MIND-BLOWING FIX:
PORTABLE BLACKOUT SHADES

Portable blackout shades (sometimes called portable blackout blinds) were one of those discoveries I wanted to shout from the rooftops. Not only did they help me sleep while visiting friends and family, but I also used them in my bedroom at home. The design is pretty simple: a 100 percent light-blocking material that attaches directly to the window glass or frame with suction cups and/or Velcro. Because they adhere directly to the glass or frame, rather than hanging a few inches in front of the window, the blinds eliminate the usual gaps that come with standard window coverings—giving you a near perfect blackout solution. If you're on a budget, you can even DIY your own. In a pinch, I've even taped black garbage bags to the window.

How-To: DIY No-Sew Portable Blackout Shades

What You'll Need
- Enough 100 percent light-blocking material to cover your window (preferably synthetic and lightweight)
- Non-damaging adhesive Velcro—for the window
- Extra-strength adhesive Velcro—for the shade (make sure it has a good hold with the non-damaging Velcro)

Instructions

1. Stick window Velcro to the corners of the glass or window frame and add additional pieces along the perimeter as needed. Get as close to the edge as possible.
2. Attach shade Velcro strips to the window Velcro strips, matching them up as closely as possible. Then peel off the adhesive backing, so the adhesive is exposed.
3. Line up your material, and stick it in place, making sure to put adequate pressure to properly adhere the shade to the Velcro, and checking to ensure the material is taut throughout. Add extra Velcro if needed to plug any light gaps.

Optional: If material isn't already cut to size, mark it while it's in place. Then remove and trim. You can also keep it oversize to be on the safe side if you want to use it on another window in the future.

4. If using for travel, bring extra Velcro to use as needed for size adjustments.

The downside to portable shades is they don't look as nice as a regular blind or shade, and you can't roll them up or down. But you can always hide them behind a more aesthetically pleasing window covering, and the big perk is you can take them with you when you travel.

THE SHOPPING FIX:
THE BLACKOUT GUIDE

If you prefer a more permanent option for blackout coverings, here are a few things to keep in mind:

Terminology

Vendors use all kinds of terms when marketing window coverings, and it can get confusing—especially since the same term can mean different things to different vendors. Whether you're shopping for shades, blinds, curtains, or drapes, for a true light-tight bedroom, *light-filtering* or *room-darkening* will not do. Look for something that's not only advertised as blackout but listed as 100 percent light-blocking. Some stores will have a special category for these, like *max blackout*. When you get home, shine a flashlight behind it to confirm you can't see through it.

You can also buy a blackout liner to hang behind non-blackout curtains. Just make sure the liner is 100 percent light-blocking.

Wraparound Rod

If using curtains or drapes, be sure you use a wraparound rod, which are now available in styles that look like regular curtain rods. This will allow you to minimize the annoying gaps between the curtain and the wall. For additional coverage, you can also use Velcro to plug any gaps. For a no-sew option, use non-damaging adhesive

Velcro on the wall and Velcro with a stronger adhesive to attach to the curtain itself.

Eva Pilgrim says she now uses a combined approach, with Velcro keeping her curtains flush to the wall, tape to prevent any gaps in between the panels, and a second curtain behind her first set to add an extra layer of light-blocking.

Side Channels or Panels

If you're using blinds or shades, there will inevitably be a small gap along the sides, which will let in some light. To block this, look for blinds or shades that come with light-blocking side channels. If you already have the blind or shade, there are several products on the market that you can purchase separately to block that light.

Alternatively, you can hang curtains over the blind or shade to give you extra coverage. Some are made extra narrow so they can be used specifically to block only the sides.

Measurements

When determining the size of your blackout curtains and installing them, make sure they come up at least three inches above the top of the window, at least three inches out from the sides of your window, and ideally all the way to the floor.

If you're using blinds or shades, make sure they're cut as accurately as possible to the width of the window to minimize the gap between the shade or blind and the window frame.

THE SURPRISING CULPRIT FIX:
DOOR BLACKOUT

Finally having my window truly blacked out with the portable shade felt like a victory in a long-running battle. But my celebration was short-lived. I quickly realized I could still see clear across the room thanks to the surprising amount of light around the doorframe. As a quick fix, I blocked the bottom of the door with a towel before going to bed, but eventually I found a more thorough and long-term solution: adhesive foam weather stripping. Just cut to size with a scissor, then peel and stick. I put it around the whole doorframe, then used a door sweep to plug the bottom. As a bonus: these also help with soundproofing.

THE FINISHING TOUCH FIX:
ELECTRICAL TAPE

With the window and door covered, I was making major progress, but still the game of whack-a-mole continued. Removing the natural light from the equation revealed how much electric light I had in my room. Alarm clocks, speakers, phone chargers—it's amazing how many devices display some kind of light.

Luckily, this one's easy: If the device can go, get it out of the room. If it has to stay, use electrical tape to block whatever light it's emitting. I was pleased to learn, the tape comes in lots of different colors, so you can make it very discreet.

THE FINISH LINE FIX:
THE HAND TESTS

In all the books and articles I've read on sleep, I found only one that addressed how to know when your room is dark enough. In his book *The Sleep Solution,* Dr. Chris Winter suggests holding your hands in front of your face. If you can see them, there's too much light.

For those who feel they don't need the room to be this dark, you can try my alternative method. Close your eyes, then repeatedly cover and uncover them with your hands. The room is dark enough when you see no difference between when your closed eyes are covered or uncovered.

THE LOGISTICAL FIX:
MOTION SENSOR STRIP LIGHTING

Even in a light-tight room you will still need to get up for a bathroom break every now and then, and we don't want anyone tripping, falling, or banging into any walls as they try to navigate their new cave. One option to be able to see where you step with minimal alerting effects is motion sensor strip lighting. As Dr. Satchin Panda explains in *The Circadian Code*, "This type of lighting is the least disruptive and will not activate the blue light sensors in your eyes." You can place it under the bed, along the floor, on stair treads—anywhere you want a little light to help you get around safely.

I actually have one of these under my side of the bed. The whole thing cost less than $20 and the setup was super easy—just stick the adhesive light strip under the bed and put the motion sensor somewhere nearby. Now when I come to bed at night, the light automatically turns on, allowing me to see clearly without getting a blast of light right before bed. And in the morning, I can see clearly without waking up my husband.

THE EVENING FIX:
MOOD LIGHTING

Despite the rewards of limiting light before bedtime, we still need to see clearly in the room as we use it throughout the evening. See chapter 8 for how to strategically use light around the house, while still limiting its potential impact on your sleep and circadian rhythm.

CHAPTER 23

Room/Bed Temperature

TEMPERATURE WAS THE MOST SURPRISING aspect of my sleep environment makeover—and it was a game changer for me when it came to sleeping through the night. But it was a frustrating road to find my solution.

Everything I read said to keep the room "cool," but what exactly that means is up for debate. Most articles say 60 to 67 degrees, others say 65 to 72, one actually says anything warmer than 60 degrees is "incorrect," and the National Sleep Foundation says "somewhere around 65." This is not only confusing but also unrealistic for those who live in warm climates.

Add to that, every time I tried to tough it out in the mid-60s, I was too cold to fall asleep and found it harder to drag myself out of bed in the morning into a cold room. At a more comfortable temperature I'd fall asleep more easily, but I'd wake up throughout the night.

The hardest part was I had no idea my wake-ups were due to temperature. Like so many people, I thought I was waking up due to stress or to go to the bathroom. And at the time, I didn't know that insomnia and temperature issues go hand in hand (see chapter 10 for more on that).

Lucky for me, my husband happened to read about something called the chiliPAD in the book *Tools of Titans* by Tim Ferriss. The chiliPAD is a mattress topper that circulates water at the temperature of your choice. In the book, several "titans" recommend it as one of their tools for success, so my husband bought it in hopes it would help me.

When we first got it, I wasn't very enthusiastic and used it inconsistently. But eventually I realized that when I remembered to turn it on, I often slept through the night. I also started realizing that when I forgot to turn it on and woke up, there was a lot of heat trapped between my body and the mattress. I'm not sure why I never noticed it before, but suddenly it was very clear—I was waking up because I was hot. I quickly stopped forgetting to turn on the chiliPAD.

Fast-forward a year and a half. We had put the chiliPAD in storage during apartment renovations, and before I had a chance to get it out, my son was born. Luckily, he started sleeping through the night relatively quickly—but I continued waking up. I assumed I'd just gotten into the habit of waking to feed him and my body needed more time to readjust. When I finally got the chiliPAD out of storage and set it back up again, the first word out of my mouth the next morning was "idiot!" I'd slept through the night for the first time in months and couldn't help but facepalm at how much of that time was probably spent awake unnecessarily.

I should mention that in general my body is not good at regulating temperature. In winter, when I get on the subway, everyone else is fine in their coats, hats, and scarves. Meanwhile I'm frantically tearing off layers out of fear I'll pass out. If I ease up on the layers, I'm absolutely freezing outside. I'm not sure why this is (my thyroid has been tested, it's fine), but I mention this because for many of you, simple, less expensive tools might do the trick.

THE GUIDELINE FIX:
WARM TO COOL

Rather than obsess over the "perfect room temperature," in his book *Sleep*, sports sleep coach Nick Littlehales offers some more practical advice: just make your bedroom slightly cooler than the rest of your home. He writes, "Whatever the temperature is, warm to cool is the mantra."

In winter, this can be as easy as cracking the bedroom window in the evening or lowering the bedroom heat. In summer, air conditioning, a fan, and/or closing bedroom window coverings to block the sun during the day can all help. If AC isn't available, Littlehales even suggests a simple DIY hack: place a few frozen water bottles in front of a fan.

But it's worth noting that you'll still want to maintain sufficient bedding to stay comfortable. As Dr. Roy Raymann tells me, the purpose of that cool bedroom air is not to make you feel cold, it's to help you feel comfortable under the covers, and less obviously—it's to give your lungs cool air to breathe, which helps cool the core.

THE SURPRISING FIX:
WARM HANDS AND FEET

Counterintuitively, another way to help drop core body temperature before bed is to gently warm your hands and feet. This kind of tricks the body into thinking you're in a warm environment and triggers a cooling response—the same cooling response that traditionally happens before sleep. Warm blood is diverted away from the core to the skin and extremities, where it can lose some of that heat to the air. Research has even shown that the degree of this heat transfer away from the core is the best physiological predictor for how quickly we'll fall asleep.

This explains why research suggests some sleep disorders may be caused by circulatory issues, common among older adults, and why narcolepsy-related sleepiness has been linked to abnormally regulated skin temperature. In an unfortunate twist, sleep loss itself can also interfere with circulation, leading to more sleep loss. But warming extremities can prove very effective at reversing that cycle. In one study, seven elderly participants who warmed their lower limbs with a heating pack saw the time it took them to fall asleep drop from a median of 47 minutes to less than 12 minutes.

What's also interesting: While Raymann says warming your hands can be as easy as running them under warm water before bed, just warming your feet might be enough. In the study mentioned above, warming the lower limbs actually resulted in warmer hands.

As for how to warm your feet, there are a number of options available. A small study on six men in South Korea found simply wearing "bed socks" (aka loose, soft socks) reduced the time it took them to fall asleep and their number of awakenings, increasing their total sleep time an average 32 minutes. If you want to step it up, the National Sleep Foundation recommends splurging on cashmere socks, adding an extra blanket on the foot of the bed, using a hot water bottle or heating pad to warm the foot of the bed before you get in, or wearing insulated slippers before bed.

But you don't want to go overboard, and as usual, you can learn from my mistake. I started my foot warming ritual with a microwavable heating pad I picked up at my local pharmacy. It was fine but very subtle. Always wanting to go the extra mile, I decided to kick things up a notch. I ordered a giant box of toe warmers—the kind sold at ski lodges—and stuck them to my socks. As I went to bed with lovely warm feet, I felt pretty smug: I was obviously a genius. But I quickly learned why the studies on this topic often use words like *gentle* heating. While the toe warmers seem to do nothing when tucked into my snowboard boots on a freezing mountain, they were a bit too effective in bed. After a little while my feet felt like they were on fire! Not exactly conducive to a good night's sleep. I went back to the heating pad.

Still, after a few weeks I felt I no longer needed the heating pad anymore. This could be because my improved sleep improved my circulation, or because entraining my circadian rhythm got my temperature rhythm back on track—or maybe a little of both.

That said, I do still sleep in socks. They're not cashmere, they're not "bed socks"—just whatever warm pair of socks I have on hand. And if anyone needs some toe warmers for their next ski trip, I've got you covered.

THE COZY FIX:
THE RIGHT BEDDING

With your core sending all that warm blood to your skin, you need to give that heat somewhere to go. Trap too much of it with your bedding and mattress and you'll obviously get too hot.

But no one ever talks about the other side of this coin. Let your skin get too cold in your newly chilled room, and you'll not only be uncomfortable, you'll actually trigger a warming response. The body protectively retains heat by drawing blood away from the skin back to the core—the opposite of ideal sleeping conditions.

I like to think of it like making a soft-boiled egg. You want your body to be slightly cool in the center (your core) but still comfortably warm on the outside (your skin, hands, and feet). As Dr. Raymann puts it, "You need to be in what is considered a sort of thermoneutral zone . . . you don't want your body to trigger any kind of countermeasure to become cool or to become warm."

Personal Bedding

In this Goldilocks scenario of needing a warm skin temp but cool core temp, our needs are very individualized—yet so many of us have two people with different temperature needs sharing the same room, the same mattress, and the same bedding. Raymann says the result is both people often compromise, "and both might not be sleeping well." He suggests that we instead look at sleep environment "from a person . . . not from a bed perspective" and, at the very least, get two different comforters or duvets. This allows each person to get the right amount of insulation for their needs and, as an added bonus, there's no fighting over the covers.

Thread Count

Despite our individualized bedding needs, all sleep experts seem to agree on one universal recommendation: bedding should be breathable. This is ironic given the current obsession with super high thread counts, which are usually not very breathable. The National Sleep Foundation recommends sticking to a thread count of between 200 and 400—enough to be soft *and* breathable.

Layers

As someone with body temperature issues, I'll add my own recommendation for bedding: layers. My husband, Tom, is from the UK, where the common setup is to sleep with just a duvet and a fitted sheet. While we were dating, I spent months struggling to get a good night's sleep at his apartment. I would wake up hot and throw the duvet off of me. But I don't like sleeping without some sort of cover, and with nothing on me, I was also a bit too cold. Eventually, I would pull the duvet back on and fall back asleep. A little while later, I'd wake up hot again. Finally, one day I had a rather comical meltdown in which I insisted that Tom "urgently" needed to get a top sheet for his bed. He agreed—out of sheer terror—and my sleep immediately improved. I finally was able to adjust my middle-of-the-night temperature spikes by sleeping just under the top sheet. Our current bed setup is pretty much the same—and I still openly threaten divorce any time Tom tries to steal the top sheet. But if we didn't have the chiliPAD, I'd add one more layer to my side of the bed to have a middle option between the top sheet and the duvet.

My friend Rosemary takes things one step further with a pillow strategy. Sleeping next to her six-five, 280-pound husband, Kevin, she's gotten used to keeping the bedroom at a cool 65 degrees. So when Kevin's not around to cuddle, she places three pillows on top of her instead. When she gets hot during the night she just rolls over, leaving the pillows on their half of the bed. "Those pillows can be more easily thrown off than my hot, sweaty, linebacker husband," she tells me, laughing. As an added bonus, she says the pillows also help her stay asleep if Kevin comes to bed late. "It's as though the disruption of him coming into bed isn't as severe if I already have the weight of the pillows on me."

So whether it's a comforter, a quilt, a top sheet, or a pillow-husband, bedding layers allow you to make quick temperature adjustments with minimal disruption to your sleep. The only downside is a few extra seconds to make the bed. Well worth it if it gives you a lot of extra minutes of quality sleep.

THE WARDROBE FIX:
THE RIGHT PAJAMAS

It's easier for the body to heat itself than to cool itself, and it's easier to throw an extra blanket on or off than it is to change your clothes in the middle of the night. So as a general rule, I recommend using extra blankets for extra warmth, and either skipping pajamas entirely or sticking to ones that are light, breathable, and if sweat is a concern, moisture-wicking. Take it from the girl who used to sleep in oversize sweats.

Also, this may sound obvious, but make sure your pj's are really comfortable. Whether it's the fabric, the fit, or some random button or tag, small irritants can be big obstacles, especially for insomniacs. So if you don't love the way it feels, don't sleep in it.

As a bonus, slipping into pajamas you love can be a great start to your bedtime routine. In her book *The Sleep Revolution,* Arianna Huffington goes so far as to call her "yummy pink pajamas" her "favorite sleep aid." She writes, "Just putting them on made me feel ready for bed—so much more so than the cotton T-shirts I usually wore. . . . they were unmistakably 'going-to-bed clothes,' not to be confused with 'going-to-the-gym clothes.' Slipping on the pj's was a signal to my body: time to shut down."

I've always aspired to be that person that has "yummy pink pajamas," but let's face it, I'm nowhere near that put-together (and to be fair, Arianna's were a gift). Still, I'm cool sleeping in cotton T-shirts, both figuratively and literally. Slipping out of my day clothes and into my soft T-shirt is a highlight of my evening and triggers that same signal: time to relax and shut down (but if anyone wants to gift me some nice pj's, I'm so here for it!).

THE MATTRESS FIX:
BED TEMP CONTROL

I can tell you from experience that if your mattress traps too much heat, ditching the covers and cranking up the AC or fan won't always cut it. Luckily there are several options to address the problem directly without buying a new bed.

Gel Pad

Believe it or not, one option I've used in a pinch is a gel pad made for dogs! The product is meant to serve as a cool surface for dogs to lie on in the summer, but when I saw it at the pet store, I thought, *Maybe that can help me too.* Sure enough, it did!

I now know they also make gel pads for humans, and several other products that work by absorbing body heat. The downside to these products is that they usually stay cool only up to three hours, so Dr. Raymann tells me they're best for someone who's too hot to fall asleep but has no trouble sleeping through the night. If the pad is big enough, you can also sleep on one half, then roll over to the other half once you feel too hot. Alternatively you can start the night with the pad next to you, then roll onto it when you feel hot, like I did.

Active Cooling or Heating

For a more long-lasting solution, Raymann recommends an active cooling/heating system, which basically means an electronic device that can keep your bed at a certain temperature all night.

Some, like the one I have, work by circulating water. Others, like the one I recently bought for my mother, circulate air through the bed. A brand called Eight Sleep even claims its products detect your heartbeat and breathing patterns and *automatically* adjust to your temperature needs throughout the night. Most of these systems offer options for half of the mattress, or the full mattress. You can even keep both sides of the mattress at two different temperatures. I use mine to keep my side of the bed comfortably cool all night, but some people also use them to preheat the bed, then turn them down or off once they get in. Whatever works for you!

My mother has pretty dramatic temperature issues, as described in chapter 10, but even she says her BedJet has helped keep her body temperature steadier, which helps her stay asleep longer.

And Eva Pilgrim credits her chiliPAD with finally allowing her to sleep through the night. She's so obsessed that the last time New York City had a blackout, Eva still found a way to get her chiliPAD running. "I used this solar battery pack that I have from hurricane coverage, and plugged that into the chiliPAD . . . And I slept through the night!" she says with a laugh.

Just be warned, a little goes a long way on the temperature dial. Almost everyone I know (including me) who has a chiliPAD froze their butt off the first few nights, thinking they needed it at 55 degrees. Mine is now set to 74 degrees, which might sound warm, but since it's so close to the skin, it's like always sleeping on the cool side of the pillow.

Unfortunately, right now these gadgets are all fairly pricey, but they're still cheaper than buying a new mattress, and have the added bonus of being semi-portable. For me, the investment wound up being worth it.

CHAPTER 24

Noise

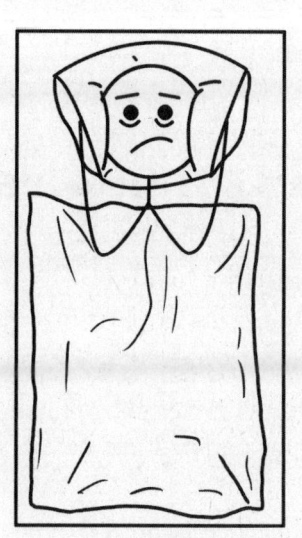

NOISE IS PROBABLY THE MOST obvious sleep disrupter. Chances are your sleep is disrupted every morning by a noisy alarm clock. But noise can also disrupt your sleep in more subtle ways.

According to a 2012 study, it's been "clearly established" that "noise events induce arousals at relatively low exposure levels." These disturbances can trigger a stress response, like elevated heart rate and blood pressure, and can pull you into lighter, less restorative, stages of sleep without fully waking you. They can also induce brief awakenings that we don't remember but that still fragment sleep. So the next day you feel tired, sleepy, moody, or otherwise crappy . . . but you don't know why.

This is especially pertinent if you live in a busy city, have a pet, or live in an apartment with paper-thin walls, ceilings, and floors that allow you to hear every move your neighbor makes (check! check! and check!).

If you're not sure if noise is affecting your sleep, try making an overnight recording (see chapter 1 for more on that). You can also just try the recommendations below to see if they help you sleep.

THE EASY-BUT-NOT-IDEAL FIX:
EARPLUGS

The easiest solution to noise is earplugs, but this falls into the same category as sleep masks for me. When I had insomnia, the mild discomfort of wearing them was still enough to disturb my sleep. Some sleep experts now tell me I just needed to find the *right* earplugs.

But Dr. Thomas Dickson, who researches how music impacts sleep, also points out that earplugs can cause wax buildup, which can lead to temporary hearing loss (until the wax buildup is removed) or ear infections, so be sure to take safe precautions against that if you do use earplugs regularly.

THE GOOD NOISE FIX:
SOUND MASKING

For me the best strategy against noise was sound masking, which is basically using soothing consistent sounds to drown out or mask the kind of sudden sounds that wake us up. Whereas earplugs reduce the volume of sounds, masking reduces the change in volume, which is ultimately what disturbs our sleep. You can do this with music, a sound machine, a fan, or any other device that makes a sound soothing enough and consistent enough for you to sleep through and loud enough to drown out other sounds that might wake you up.

Music

I find music to be the most interesting of the sound-masking tools because it actually carries additional sleep-promoting properties, so much so that Dr. Dickson says "it can turn severe insomnia into moderate insomnia" and "it can turn people with mild insomnia into healthy sleepers."

But to get these results, Dickson says music needs to be used at the same time every night for at least thirty days. And it's common not to see significant results in the first week. He says this is where many insomniacs give up on music and miss out on its benefits. "Music is a bit like working out, in that when you work out, you suddenly just don't have a six-pack the next day," he says. "With music, the more you use music as a sleep aid over time, the more effective it becomes."

Trevor Ault tells me he's been using this technique for years with his own sleep playlist. "It's eight songs, all but one of them are instrumental so that I don't get distracted by the words, and they're in the same order," he tells me. Trevor's even loaded the playlist to his Amazon Echo, so he doesn't have to look at any screens to turn it on. "I can just say, 'Alexa, it's bedtime,' and it will tell me the weather for the next morning. Then, I'm a moron, so I make it say 'Good night, boss' to me, and then it plays the playlist," he says, laughing.

Contrary to Dickson's recommendations, Trevor doesn't use his playlist at the same time every day, because his work and sleep schedule vary a bit, but he still thinks the playlist has had a positive impact on his sleep. "It helps relax me. I think it's worked enough," he says.

For those who want to use music for sound masking, Dickson recommends music that includes high-, medium-, and low-pitched sounds being played at the same time. Otherwise, if your music has only low-pitched sounds, a sudden high-pitched sound can still easily disturb your sleep and vice versa. Alternatively, Dickson says "music combined with nature sounds is also an option and has been used successfully in sleep studies."

That said, there's no research examining the impact on sleep from listening to music throughout the entire night. So music might best be used on a sleep timer to help initiate sleep rather than for sound masking all night.

Interestingly, Dickson also says for musicians, like me, music isn't always the best choice because we tend to listen to it in a more analytical way, so music is likely to make our brain more active. "You might listen to changes in harmony, key changes, sophisticated changes in rhythm," he says. "And for those reasons, it might not be the best sleep aid for you."

Colored Noise

The most effective sound for sound masking is white noise or colored noise. True white noise, the most familiar of these sounds, is essentially all sound frequencies a human can hear played at the same volume, which sounds a lot like TV or radio static. But while white noise is the one most frequently recommended in sleep literature, Dickson tells me humans hear lower frequencies as quieter, so some, like me, find white noise to be too high-pitched and irritating. Obviously, feeling irritated is not ideal for sleep.

Instead, Dickson suggests pink noise, which is a kind of white noise with reduced higher frequencies; gray noise, which is similar to pink noise but engineered to specifically match how we hear; or brown noise, which is like pink or gray noise with the bass turned up even higher. But he cautions against using a phone for this. "Mobile phones don't have the low-frequency sounds, so if you're using a mobile phone for masking, you're not going to have the effect of pink noise or brown noise," he tells me. Instead Dickson recommends using a separate speaker, headband headphones (mentioned below), or an actual sound machine.

Nature Sounds

Another option for sound masking is nature sounds, like rainfall or a rushing river. Dickson says compared to white or colored noise, nature sounds "might not be as good at masking unpleasant background sounds because they don't fill the entire frequency spectrum." But he says nature sounds do still provide decent masking benefits and carry the extra bonus of promoting relaxation and reducing "anxiety, agitation, and a lot of these kinds of things that are associated with insomnia." This is my personal preference if I'm in a scenario where I need decent sound masking.

Fan

Since I no longer sleep during the day, I no longer need robust sound masking. I also want to be sure I hear my son if he cries in the middle of the night. But I still like some ambient noise while I sleep. So instead of nature sounds or colored noise, I just turn on the small fan on my nightstand.

Dickson says there's currently no research on using an air conditioner or fan for sound masking, but he says he believes these would be well suited to sound masking because they cover a wide spectrum of sound and anecdotally many people enjoy sleeping to that sound. As for whether they'd produce the same feelings of pleasantness and relaxation as nature sounds, Dickson says there's no way to know without a study, but he suggests some may find them more pleasant than colored noise.

Deciding between these categories will come down to your individual needs and preferences. Just be sure your sound masking isn't so loud that you risk damaging your hearing or sleeping through the fire alarm. Dickson suggests a maximum of 30 decibels.

THE DO-NOT-DISTURB FIX:
HEADPHONE HEADBAND

If you're a fan of sound masking or any other audio at bedtime, but your partner isn't, headphone headbands are a cost-effective way to comfortably listen to audio while you sleep without disturbing anyone around you. And they also have the additional benefit of reducing your ability to hear unwanted noise. My SleepPhones even helped me sleep during the day despite a neighbor's construction project.

There are also earbuds advertised specifically for use while sleeping, but like with ear plugs, Dickson warns to take precautions against earwax buildup if you decide to go this route.

As when choosing a sleep mask, test out different brands or models to see what's most comfortable for you.

THE PHONE FIX:
DO NOT DISTURB SETTING

After creating your silent oasis, the last thing you want is to have it all undone because someone butt-dialed you. I set my phone to automatically go on "Do Not Disturb" every night and automatically go back into regular mode in the morning. This means I don't have to remember to silence and un-silence it every day, which I definitely won't. More importantly, you can set "Do Not Disturb" to ring for certain numbers or to ring if someone calls twice in a row, which means I can sleep soundly knowing I won't be disturbed for no reason but that my loved ones or work can still reach me in an emergency.

THE BONUS FIX:
BLACKOUT + SOUNDPROOFING

If you've blacked out your room with the tools listed in chapter 22, you're already ahead of the game. Window coverings, weather stripping, and door sweeps don't just block light, they also help to block sound, making your room both darker *and* quieter.

CHAPTER 25

Snoring/Sleep Apnea Solutions

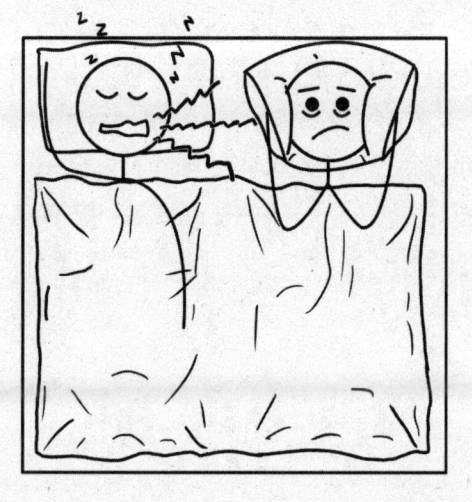

SNORING IS OFTEN THOUGHT OF as a sleep environment issue because sharing a bedroom with someone who snores loudly can make it nearly impossible to sleep—especially if you have your own sleep problems. But what often goes undiscussed is that snoring can also disturb the sleep of the person doing the snoring. Studies have shown that compared to people who don't snore, snorers are substantially more likely to experience excessive daytime sleepiness or decreased daytime alertness, as well as other medical issues—even if they don't have sleep apnea.

While it's still not clear why that is, Dr. Jordan Stern tells me that snoring "could be causing brain arousal." Since insomniacs are more prone to arousal, this can be even more problematic if you're a snoring insomniac.

So whether it's for your partner's sake, your sake, or both, if you snore, the tools below can help you to identify what's causing your snoring and, more importantly, how you can fix it.

THE AS-YOU-GO FIX:
RECORD AND MONITOR YOURSELF

As you try the suggestions below, record yourself at night, then use your sleep diary to track how each tool impacts your snoring. You can also use an app like SnoreLab to easily record yourself and monitor your progress in one place.

THE NASAL FIX:
OPEN YOUR NOSE

While it often sounds like snoring comes from the nose, snoring actually comes from the throat, but the nose can play a critical role in snoring if it's congested. As Dr. Jordan Stern explains, "If you cannot breathe through your nose and you have to breathe through your mouth . . . you have to open your mouth and you have to drop your jaw." This narrows the throat and leads to snoring.

Nasal Strips

One way to help facilitate nose breathing during sleep is with nasal strips, which adhere to the outside of the nose and help to open the nasal passages. I find nasal strips to be especially helpful to my sleep if I'm dealing with nasal congestion—no more waking up because my nose is clogged. And I find that the ability to sleep better helps me kick whatever's causing the nasal congestion much faster.

Stern says the efficacy of nasal strips will vary person to person because "everybody's got different nasal anatomy." So this may not work for everyone, but it's an easy and affordable thing to try. There are also a few nasal dilators on the market, like the Mute or NasalAid, that claim to perform a similar function but are reusable.

Nose Cones

If your problem area is more in the nostrils, rather than in the upper part of the nasal passage, Stern says nasal cones might help. These are small ventilated cone-shaped devices that are inserted into the nostrils to help open the bottom of the nasal passages.

Nasal Spray

To test if a nasal spray will help your sleep and snoring, Stern recommends starting with an over-the-counter oxymetazoline nasal spray (aka Afrin). The good thing about this kind of spray is it takes effect within just minutes. The downside is these sprays can have side effects, and the body can also become dependent on them. So Stern suggests using oxymetazoline for only one or two nights, an hour before bed and "if that works, then you can go to a nonaddictive spray, such as Flonase." Stern says a nasal steroid like Flonase can take a few days to kick in but is safe for long-term use. Still, be sure to check with your doctor before trying any nasal spray.

If none of these suggestions work to alleviate your nasal congestion, see an ear, nose, and throat specialist, as you may have a deviated septum, polyps, or another issue that can be resolved only by a medical professional.

THE SIDEWAYS FIX:
SLEEP POSITION

You've probably already heard that sleeping on your back is the worst position for snoring. That's because when you're on your back, your jaw drops and pushes your tongue into your throat. But did you know there's a best position for snoring?

Sleep on Your Side

Sleep experts seem to agree that the best position for sleep, especially to avoid snoring, is the side position. Dr. Stern says, "In general, the left side position is better because it also decreases the incidence of acid reflux," which not only disturbs sleep but can also lead to snoring by causing swelling in the throat or nose.

Based on sleep studies he's reviewed, Sterns says it's quite common for patients to think they're sleeping on their side when they actually spend half the night on their back. For those who want to ensure they stay on their side, Stern says you can consider various products marketed to keep you from rolling onto your back, or you can go with a DIY solution: sew a tennis ball to the back of your sleeping shirt.

Sniffing Position

Many people find sleeping on their back to be most comfortable, so they instead try to mitigate snoring by using extra pillows. But Stern tells me this often backfires, because by lifting the head, "you're actually going to close your airway . . . your neck is flexed so that your chin is touching your chest. That's the worst breathing position possible."

Instead, Stern says if you're going to sleep on your back, you should place your pillow or pillows under your neck and shoulders, so your head is in the so-called sniffing position. This is when your chin is out and up—as if you're trying to sniff something slightly in front of you. Stern says another way to ensure correct positioning is to "put your hands on your head . . . and then raise your chin." This position straightens the airway, minimizing the chance for snoring.

For snorers on the hunt for the perfect pillow, Stern says search for one that puts you into the sniffing position, and if you sleep on your back, you might also consider a pillow under your shoulders to help encourage that sniffing position as much as possible.

THE ELEVATED FIX:
BED WEDGE

Another useful tool recommended to combat snoring and acid reflex is a wedge pillow, which keeps your upper body at a slight incline rather than completely flat. This not only helps better positioning of the airway but also makes it harder for acid to travel up the esophagus and give you reflux.

THE FEEL LIKE AN ATHLETE FIX:
MOUTH GUARD

An anti-snoring mouth guard or night guard is a great solution, not just for snoring, but also for obstructive sleep apnea. Stern says a custom-fit appliance created by a medical professional is the most comfortable and effective option. It's also covered by most insurance for those diagnosed with sleep apnea. Just make sure you go to a provider that takes insurance.

However, for those who don't have the option to go through insurance or don't want to go through the process of having a custom appliance made, Stern says so-called boil-and-bite options can also work. Unlike custom mouth guards, which are tailor-made to fit your mouth, boil-and-bite mouth guards are a standard shape but become malleable when heated. So you put them in boiling water, then bite into them to mold them to the shape of your mouth.

For those going this route, Stern says look for a boil-and-bite mouth guard that is as small as possible, for comfort reasons; and more importantly, make sure it's adjustable, meaning you can gradually adjust the position of the jaw forward. If it works but is uncomfortable, Stern strongly recommends a custom appliance, "because you know that it will work but it will be much more comfortable."

THE SHUT IT FIX:
CHIN STRAP/MOUTH TAPE

If mouth guards just aren't for you, Stern says some might find success using a chin strap at night. This won't protrude the jaw forward like a snoring mouth guard will, but it will keep the jaw from dropping. For some, that may be enough.

Believe it or not, there are also lots of different mouth tape products that do exactly what they sound like: they tape your mouth shut so you keep your jaw closed and have to breathe through your nose. For comfort reasons, Stern prefers the chin strap method to mouth tape, but anecdotally some people swear by mouth tape products. And these products do claim to be specially designed for comfort and painless removal. (*Do not* just slap some tape from your hardware drawer on your mouth!) Some might also prefer mouth tape to a chin strap, as it doesn't require any straps around the head, which are especially annoying if you have long hair. Try whichever sounds more comfortable for you!

THE SOBERING FIX:
AVOID LATE ALCOHOL/MUSCLE RELAXERS

You might notice your snoring worsens or only happens after a night of drinking. That's because one of alcohol's functions is to relax your muscles. This may help you fall asleep, but unfortunately it also relaxes the muscles in the throat and causes snoring. Alcohol also relaxes our esophageal valves, which causes acid reflux . . . which also causes snoring. The same is true for other muscle relaxers as well.

This doesn't mean you can never enjoy a drink, but it's another reason to enjoy that drink earlier, giving yourself enough time to sober up before bedtime. (See chapter 15 for more on how alcohol impacts sleep.)

THE GOES-BOTH-WAYS FIX:
WEIGHT LOSS

For someone who snores due to excess weight, weight loss can actually be not just a treatment but a *cure* for snoring and sleep apnea. The problem is, as Stern points out, "It's very difficult to lose weight if you have untreated sleep apnea." So while weight loss can cure your sleep apnea, you may find it helpful to first treat your sleep apnea, so you can achieve that weight loss more easily. Stern says sometimes as little as five pounds can make all the difference.

THE SIDE EFFECT FIX:
AVOID ACID REFLUX

It's commonly known that acid reflux, which happens when stomach acid travels up the esophagus, can disturb your sleep. But Stern says what often goes unaddressed is that that acid can cause swelling of the throat, the sinuses, and the uvula, that "little punching bag in the back of the throat." He says the coughing and throat clearing that often accompanies acid reflux can also contribute to swelling. And all that swelling can then cause or worsen snoring. The worst part: The snoring itself can irritate the uvula, making the swelling worse . . . which can make the snoring worse.

As for how to avoid reflux, *Dropping Acid: The Reflux Diet Cookbook & Cure*, coauthored by Stern, lays out the best and worst foods for a reflux sufferer. Stern also advises having your last meal at least three hours before bed. But if, like me, you can't sleep on an empty stomach, you might be better off having a reflux-friendly snack one to two hours before bed, as failing to sleep because you're hungry can also lead to reflux. (See chapter 18 for more on that.)

THE ALLERGY FIX:
POLLEN PROTECTION

One key reason our nose gets congested is allergies, especially to pollen. But while you might think this happens as a result of inhaling pollen through the nose, that's only one way pollen reaches our sinuses. Stern says think of pollen more like a respiratory virus. Everything we learned about how to avoid getting Covid-19—do the same to avoid pollen during allergy season.

Glasses/Sunglasses

Counterintuitively, one way to keep pollen from getting into your sinuses is by wearing glasses or sunglasses—preferably big ones. "Pollen gets into your nose through the eyes because . . . that tear duct goes into the nose," Stern explains. So protecting your eyes can in turn protect your nose.

Shower/Bath Before Bed

While glasses can block pollen from getting in your eyes, they won't prevent it from getting in your hair. "If you haven't taken a shower before you go to sleep and rinsed all the pollen out of your hair, you're taking pollen into your bed," Stern says. The simple solution: wash your hair before going to bed.

Nasal Rinse

While you're washing your hair, give your nose a rinse too, or use a nasal rinse before bed to clear pollen from your sinuses. Stern says this effect of clearing out pollen is actually the main reason nasal rinses are effective for those with sinus or nasal issues.

AC vs. Open Windows

While open windows may be better for the environment, Stern says closed windows are better for your allergies. If that means turning on the air conditioning, make sure your filters are clean, as a dirty air conditioning filter can also aggravate allergies.

THE MARGINAL FIX:
AVOID SALT

Have you ever noticed that after having a very salty meal you wake up with bags under your eyes? This is because excessive salt causes our body to retain water, which can cause puffiness in certain areas. Dr. Stern says once you lie down, that puffiness can affect the throat and nose, which can cause or worsen snoring. Thus lowering salt intake can decrease snoring or apnea, as shown in a 2018 study, though the study shows the impact is "limited."

THE PROFESSIONAL FIX:
GET A SLEEP STUDY

If none of these remedies work, see a sleep specialist, preferably one who's also an ear, nose, and throat specialist. They can evaluate you for sleep apnea and other sleep disorders and explore additional options like CPAP, Inspire, or surgery.

CHAPTER 26

Mattress/Pillow

OF ALL THE THINGS THAT make up your sleep environment, the most important, or at least the most expensive, is usually the surface you're sleeping on. Yet for the amount of time and money we spend on our mattress, too many of us are flying blind when it comes to knowing what's best. That's partly because, despite what some mattress companies would have us believe, there is no one best mattress. Instead, what constitutes an ideal mattress is very personal and depends on a long list of factors, including body type, body weight, body temperature, and sleeping position.

Sleep experts will often just say to pick out one that's "comfortable," but what feels comfortable for a few minutes in a store, when a salesperson is standing over you, isn't always what's comfortable long term—especially if you don't know what to look for.

So if you're in the market for a new mattress, the tools below can help guide you on a few main points—and if you don't want a new mattress, you'll also find ways to upgrade your current one.

That said, while a good mattress setup can help ensure we have a comfortable night's sleep, unless your sleep problems are obviously caused by your mattress, a mattress makeover is not going to fix them. Instead, you'll have to address what's causing your sleep problems, which is likely covered in part 1, 2, or 3 of this book. Then make your mattress adjustments as a finishing touch.

THE VISUAL FIX:
THE LINE TEST

The most basic function of a mattress is a simple but often over-looked one: to keep our body properly aligned while we sleep. No matter how great the mattress feels when you first lie on it, if it doesn't give you the right amount of support and cushioning, it will not be comfortable long term. It may even cause you pain.

So whether you're analyzing a new mattress or your current one, instead of just gauging how it feels, the line test will help you gauge how it supports you.

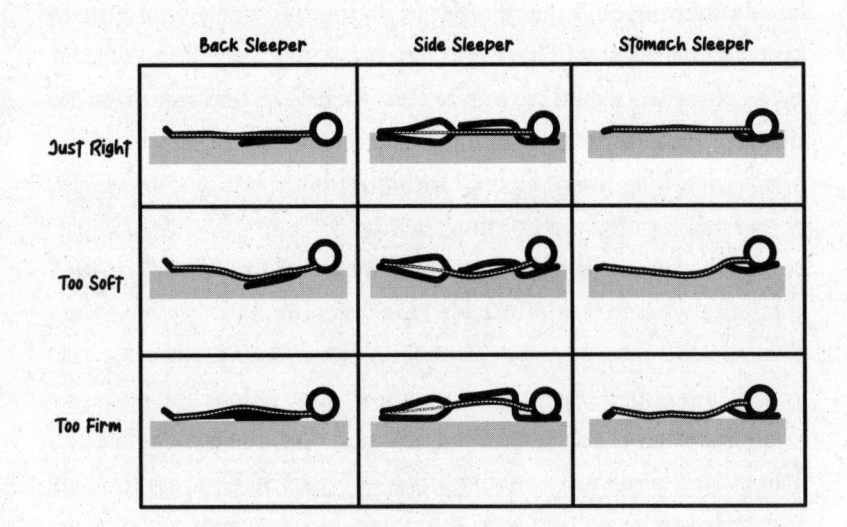

How-To: The Line Test

1. Position a camera level to the mattress so you can photograph yourself lying on it from the side, or recruit someone to help you.
2. Lie on the bare mattress in your favorite sleeping position(s), with no pillow (side sleepers can put a hand under their head if needed). Use a timer or your recruit to photograph yourself.

3.   Draw an imaginary line along your spine, from the center of your
     head through the center of your torso and through to the center of
     your knees.
4.   Assuming your bed is flat:

     •   If the line is fairly straight, as if you're standing with good
         posture, your bed is giving you the right amount of support and
         cushioning.
     •   If the line curves downward at your midsection, then back up
         through your legs, the mattress is not firm enough.
     •   If the line curves upward at your midsection, then back down
         toward your legs, the mattress is not soft enough.

The one caveat to all this is that some people with certain back or
neck issues may do better on an extra-firm mattress. Neurosurgeon
Dr. Paul Young tells me, for his patients with these kinds of issues,
he recommends a mattress that's extra firm with no pillow top layer.
So as always, don't let the advice above interfere with following the
advice of your doctor.

THE FEELING FIX:
PRESSURE POINTS

Another way to gauge if a mattress is giving you the right amount
of support and cushioning is to feel for any uneven pressure points.
Depending on your sleep position, you'll feel these on your head,
ear, shoulder, hip, pelvis, knees, and/or feet. "When you're not
aligned, generally people don't notice the curvature or the sagging
of the spine. They'll notice, 'oh, my hips hurt after a while, because
the surface is too hard to allow my hip to sink into it,'" Dr. Chris
Winter tells me.

But you won't feel that pain right away, so test the mattress for at
least fifteen minutes, and look for more subtle signs.

I compare this to shoe shopping. Have you ever tried on a shoe and it feels fine at first? Then you actually wear the shoe for a while and realize it digs into your ankle, your heel hurts, and your pinkie toe is begging for mercy. After doing this enough times, I try to be much more aware now when trying things on. The question isn't "Is this causing me pain right now?" Instead it's "Do I feel any pressure that might cause me discomfort after a while?" If the answer is yes, the shoe doesn't fit. The same goes for the mattress.

THE HARD FIX:
THE FLOOR TEST

If you're debating whether a firmer mattress will be better for you, there is a free tool at your disposal: the floor. Dr. Young recommends putting a comforter over a carpeted surface and sleeping on that for a few days. This way you can test if you feel better on a firmer surface before buying a new mattress or adjusting your current one. Young says patients typically report success or failure after three or four nights.

THE TOO FIRM FIX:
ADDING SOFTNESS

If you've decided your mattress is too firm, a mattress topper is a quick, effective, and fairly affordable fix. As someone who's had several mattress toppers, I'm always surprised at how dramatically they can transform an overly firm mattress into a cloud of comfort.

If only one partner wants more cushion, you can even add the topper to only half of the bed. You can also try rotating or flipping the mattress to see if that helps.

THE TOO SOFT FIX:
ADDING FIRMNESS

If your bed isn't giving you enough support, start by checking the foundation. Is any part of the box spring or platform squeaking, sagging, or broken?

Even if all looks fine, replacing or topping a box spring or slats with a piece of plywood can help make the mattress on top of it more supportive. If only one partner wants more support, you can even do this to only half of the bed. My husband and I added plywood over our own bed slats years ago and were pleasantly surprised at how dramatically that changed the feel of the mattress.

You can also try rotating or flipping the mattress to see if that helps.

THE HEAD FIX:
PICKING A PILLOW

To borrow an analogy from sports sleep coach Nick Littlehales, a pillow is like an insole for a mattress. Just like you might use an insole to get a little more arch support for your foot or to make a loose shoe a bit more snug, pillows are there to fill small gaps and keep our body aligned where our mattress falls short. For most of us, our pillow should keep our head in the same position as when we stand with good posture. The exception to this is snorers who sleep on their backs in the sniffing position detailed in chapter 25.

In general, back sleepers and stomach sleepers should need little to no pillow support, compared to side sleepers, who need a bit more to fill the gap between your shoulder and your cheek. Some side sleepers might also find added comfort in placing a small pillow between their knees or hugging a body pillow or king-size pillow.

This was especially helpful to me during pregnancy, and I still sleep hugging my king-size pillow. Sorry, hubs.

But Littlehales says if your mattress is providing you with the right amount of support, even side sleepers should need no more than one flat hand to put their head in alignment, and back and stomach sleepers should need no pillow at all, though they can use a very shallow one if they prefer.

If you find yourself gravitating toward thick pillows or stacking more than one, go back and do the line test, detailed earlier in this chapter. Chances are your mattress support is off or your current pillow setup is giving your head too much support and throwing your head out of alignment.

In addition, in his book *The One-Week Insomnia Cure,* Dr. Jason Ellis recommends an easy pillow test: Hold the pillow out in front of you lengthwise. If it bends in half, "it is dead and it is time for a replacement."

THE SPACE FIX:
GO BIG OR GO DOUBLE

Finding a mattress with perfect support will help only so much if you and your partner are constantly kicking or rolling into each other all night. Littlehales' advice: Buy the biggest mattress you can afford. "If you have got a regular sleeping partner, then you want as much space for you to be able to sleep as an individual, as a human, as possible, so that you can reduce the impacts of having somebody next door," he tells me.

But, since we all have different needs from a mattress, Dr. Roy Raymann suggests taking this one step further: skip the king mattress and instead put two standard twin XL mattresses side by side. They occupy the same amount of space, so you can put them on a regular king-size frame and use regular king-size sheets. But this way you can each enjoy a mattress picked specifically for your needs, rather than settling for something that's just okay for both of you. This is especially helpful for partners who have very different weights, body types, or sleeping positions. Having two mattresses also reduces your chances of feeling your partner's movements on your side of the bed.

If you do go this route, try to get two mattresses with uniform thickness, so they still look like one mattress, and be sure they're the standard 38 inches across. You can also get a bed bridge, to eliminate the gap in between.

Alternatively you can look for one mattress that offers different firmness options for each half.

If you find it particularly disruptive to share a sleeping space with your partner, you can also opt to sleep in different rooms for a while. (More on that in the next chapter.)

THE TEMPERATURE FIX:
INSULATION LEVEL

Those of us who've woken up feeling like our bed was giving us a tan know mattress temperature can make a huge difference in our sleep. Unfortunately, how much heat your mattress will trap is not something you can sense in a typical in-store mattress test, even if you take your time.

In general, foam mattresses tend to trap more heat than innerspring mattresses. But Dr. Roy Raymann says the manufacturer should be able to tell you whether the mattress has a high or low insulation level. Those who want a cooler bed should aim for something with a low insulation factor. Those who want something warmer should go with a higher insulation factor. He says you should also ask about ventilation and research the material the mattress is made of. "Latex has a higher insulation factor, for instance, compared to most of the foams, and definitely more than a spring mattress," he tells me.

If you find your current mattress is too hot or too cool, Raymann also recommends products that offer active cooling or active heating, rather than passive options like a mattress topper with a cooling gel. "Your body will easily warm those phase change materials that are on there. And then it's just warm," he tells me. (See more on temperature in chapters 10 and 23.)

THE BUYER'S REMORSE FIX:
RETURN POLICY

To ensure you don't get stuck with the wrong mattress, perhaps the most important thing to look out for is the return policy. A few crucial questions: How long is the trial period? Does the company pick up the mattress or do you have to ship it back? At what cost? Do they charge a restocking fee?

"It's really nice to have an exit strategy that's not 'pack this thing up yourself and take it to a UPS drop-off point,'" Dr. Chris Winter tells me. "I think a lot of people have been like, 'Well, this isn't perfect, but my God, I don't want to go through the schlepp of taking it back.'" Some customizable mattresses also come with the option to exchange specific parts to increase firmness or softness—which is far easier than shipping back the entire mattress.

CHAPTER 27

Sharing

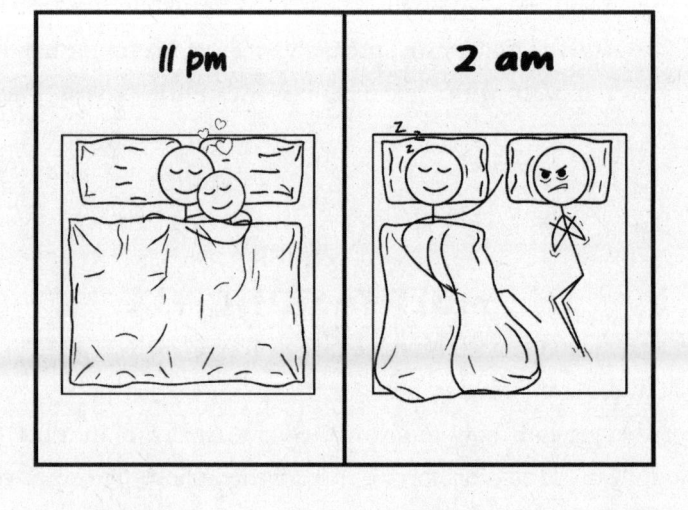

OF ALL THE THINGS IN your sleep environment, the one you probably have the least control over is the person you share it with. There are few things more frustrating for someone with sleep issues than to finally fall asleep only to be woken up by a stray leg, a stolen blanket, a light turning on . . . or any of the countless ways our partners can disrupt our sleep.

When this would happen to me, my internal (and sometimes external) monologue would immediately fire up: *That's it, I'm totally screwed! We all know I can't fall asleep once I wake up. Now I'm going to be exhausted, AGAIN!* The more I would focus on this, the angrier I would get at my husband: *He knows I can't fall back asleep. Why would he (insert whatever minor thing he did to wake me)?!* Of course all this ruminating on how upset I was and how hard it would be for me to fall back asleep only made it more certain that I wouldn't.

As hard as it is, the better way to handle these disruptions is to try not to dwell on them—or on your momentary disdain for your spouse. If you're frustrated that you can't fall back asleep, instead leave the bed, go do something enjoyable and relaxing, and come back when you feel sleepy again.

Of course, the much more preferable scenario is to not have the disruption to begin with. The Fixes below can help prevent them.

THE MULTITASKING FIX:
ROOM ZONES

Before we get into how to arrange your room for more than one person, I wanted to offer some quick advice on how to arrange your room for more than one function.

Sleep literature often dictates that we should use our bedroom only for sleep and sex so that our brain can form a clear association between entering that room and being sleepy and relaxed. But while it would be great if we could all turn our bedrooms into the "sleep oasis" so many articles recommend, doing so will not cure your sleep disorder, as some of these articles ridiculously suggest.

Having one room dedicated entirely to sleep also is just not realistic for a lot of people—including me. My husband currently works from home and I do most of my writing from home, so we need a workspace. But we live in a city apartment and don't have a spare room. The only logical place for our mini-office setup is in our bedroom. And guess what? We still sleep fine.

The key is to not get too fixated on these things and just draw as much of a distinction as possible between when and where you do wakeful activities and when and where you sleep. Our bedroom, for example, has all the office stuff in one corner—you could call that our "work zone" within the room. Our bed, meanwhile, is up against the opposite wall, which is also a different color than the rest of the room—a "sleep zone," if you will. We also try not to leave evidence of unfinished work on the desk, so that we're not reminded of that as we're going to sleep. This can also apply to unfolded clothes or any other bedroom clutter. If it doesn't bother you, fine, but if it stresses you out, try to get it out of sight, especially at bedtime.

For the same reason, if kids play in their bedrooms, pediatric sleep experts often advise having a designated play area away from the bed and putting toys away at night so kids aren't overly stimulated as they try to sleep.

If you're in a scenario where you have to do non-sleeping activities, like watching TV or doing homework, on the bed itself, you may find it helpful to make the bed look different during this time—like putting a different-colored blanket on it during the day. This way your brain sees the blanket as a sign that it's wake time, and the bed without that blanket as a cue that it's time to sleep.

THE SHARED BED FIX:
DIVIDE AND CONQUER

When my former director Sandy Panfel celebrated his thirty-fifth wedding anniversary, I asked him what the secret was to a long-lasting marriage. I expected him to say something like "open communication" or "never go to bed angry." Instead, without any pause, he held two fingers up, looked me dead in the eye, and said, "Two comforters."

Sandy and his wife had clearly accepted and leaned into what so many long-term couples are afraid to admit: while we love to cuddle when we're awake, sleep time is a different story. "We like the partnership, the sex, the spooning, the security of waking up in the morning and there's your partner," sports sleep coach Nick Littlehales tells me. "But generally, when anybody goes to sleep, they will turn away from their partner, create their own little space, and 'I'll see you in the morning.'"

If this sounds familiar, it can be helpful to think of a bed as two sleep zones rather than one shared sleeping surface. As explained in chapter 26, one way to facilitate this is by getting the biggest bed you can afford and fit in your room, or two twin XL mattresses on one king frame, each chosen to suit their respective sleeper.

If you're not in the market for a new mattress, you can also customize the firmness and softness of each side of your current mattress with plywood and/or a mattress topper. This process is also described in chapter 26.

To top off your two-zoned mattress, Dr. Roy Raymann recommends two comforters or duvets instead of one. This allows each sleeper to choose a comforter that suits their temperature needs, and it also means no more being woken up by a spontaneous game of blanket tug-of-war. If your spouse somehow transforms from a normal human at night to one whose superpower is radiating heat like the sun—not naming any names—then separate bedding can also help prevent their body heat from making you overheat.

You can also add an extra blanket on one side of the bed and just use it as a decorative throw blanket during the day, or if you want to splurge, look into active cooling or active heating options, which are available for just one side of the bed or in dual-zoned options. (More on that in chapter 23.)

THE DIFFERENT BEDTIMES FIX:
CUDDLE TIME

When a couple is made up of an early bird and a night owl, they often still default to going to bed at the same time. Unless they've shifted their circadian rhythm, this usually means the night owl is going to bed before they're naturally sleepy, which can lead to insomnia.

But for some, going to bed at different times might feel a bit too impersonal. So Dr. Jason Ellis recommends creating a cuddle time, where you go to bed together at the early bird's bedtime and cuddle in bed for roughly fifteen to twenty minutes (or however long works best for you). The key is that the night owl should not intend to go to sleep yet. This time is exclusively to enjoy some closeness with your partner. Then you can leave the bedroom and go about your evening routine until you're ready for sleep. If you prefer to shift your circadian rhythms to more closely match each other, check out part 3 for more on that.

THE DO-NOT-DISTURB FIX:
PARTNER SIGHTS/SOUNDS

Blacking out and soundproofing your room will be only so helpful if the source of the light or sound disturbing you is coming from your partner.

My husband and I recently tackled this when I started anchoring for *ABC News Live*. The new job gives me the closest to normal hours I've ever had, and the perks of that are endless. But one downside: my husband is now in lighter stages of sleep as I get ready for work compared to when I was waking up in the middle of the night, which means his sleep is more easily disturbed.

Underbed Light

I tried to avoid disturbing Tom by using my phone flashlight to get around the room in the morning, but that was still bright enough to wake him. After some troubleshooting, we found a solution: a motion-activated strip light that you stick to the bottom of the bed (or wherever you want to put it). The whole thing cost less than twenty bucks. Now as soon as I step down from the bed, the floor light automatically turns on. This allows me to see clearly, but because the light is soft and aimed at the floor, it doesn't disturb my husband. Problem solved. As I explained in chapter 22, this also allows me to navigate my room at night without having to turn on any disruptive bright lights. Everybody wins!

Sleep Mask Tips

While my underbed light doesn't disturb my husband, I'm not sure the same would be true if our roles were reversed. When I worked the overnight shift, it never failed that the second he opened our bedroom door in the morning to tiptoe out, the light from the living room would wake me. I'm lucky that I was able to solve this problem by moving into the guest room for a while (more on that later), but if we didn't have that option, I now feel confident I could have made it work with a sleep mask.

Still, sleep masks aren't the no-brainer they sometimes sound like. For starters, you have to find the right sleep mask. (See chapter 22 for more on that.)

It's also important to note the arousal that fuels insomnia can also make us more sensitive to things like light and sound—but also touch. So we might be disturbed more easily by the sensation of wearing something like an eye mask. This is yet another reason it's important to address bedtime arousal through the methods in parts 2 and 3 of this book.

Partner Sounds

Addressing arousal should also make earplugs more tolerable, and I'm told that with some trial and error anyone can find earplugs that are comfortable enough to sleep in, including custom options if needed. Still, I prefer to use sound masking to drown out partner sounds and, if needed, a headphone headband. Both are detailed in chapter 25.

Snoring

If you or your partner is disturbing the other's sleep by snoring, the suggestions above will help, but the much better solution is to address the snoring itself. This is especially true since snoring can present problems far worse than the noise disruption. So, if you or your partner snores, please, please, please, read chapter 25.

THE FURRY FIX:
PETS

I'll keep this part short. While many of us love to cuddle with our fur babies, most pets have very different circadian rhythms and sleep patterns than humans do. That means they're likely to be moving around when we're trying to sleep. This especially true for cats, who are more nocturnal than dogs. Pets can also bring allergens into the bed, which can cause or worsen snoring and other breathing issues.

If you're going to invite your pet into your room or bed, do so only if you think it's really worth having your sleep disrupted throughout the night. And at the very least, if they wear a jingly collar during the day or anything else that makes noise, remove it before you go to bed.

THE SPLIT FIX:
SLEEP DIVORCE

While there are many ways to troubleshoot the obstacles a bed partner may pose, for some there's no better solution than just moving to separate beds or separate rooms—aka a sleep divorce.

The National Sleep Foundation's 2005 Sleep in America poll found that 23 percent of respondents who lived with their partner reported sleeping in a separate bed or bedroom or on the couch. This might sound like a relationship-ending move, but for many couples the experience can be very positive.

One of those couples is my colleague, Dan Harris, and his wife, Bianca. As Dan explains, "She would wake me up if she came in later and I was already asleep, and then I'd wake up and be furious. Or our kid wakes up a lot in the middle of the night and will only accept her. So every time she wakes up in the middle of the night, I wake up, and I'm pissed." On the flip side, Dan says he often goes to the bathroom overnight and also moves a lot in his sleep, both of which would wake up Bianca. "We were disturbing each other's sleep a lot," he says.

But the obstacles of sharing a bed can go beyond physical disturbances. Dan, for example, takes comfort in knowing that if he can't sleep, he can just read for fifteen to twenty minutes and that will "knock him out." He also likes to know he can move around in bed if needed. And of course we all like to know we can go to the bathroom when nature calls. But with Bianca in the room, Dan couldn't do any of that without waking her. "I felt trapped," he says.

This feeling is arguably much more powerful than someone physically waking you, because the main thing that drives insomnia is worry. Now, because we love our partner, we're worried not only about our own sleep but also about disturbing *their* sleep. There's also a new consequence in the mix: "If I don't manage to fall asleep, I'm going to be stuck in this bed all night, unable to even move!"

By putting more pressure on ourselves, we increase our performance anxiety around sleep, thus making it harder to sleep. Do this long enough and you end up with chronic insomnia.

I'm lucky that my husband is a pretty heavy sleeper and tends to fall asleep very easily. He always went out of his way to assure me not to worry about disturbing his sleep when I was struggling with my own. But we still had our own temporary sleep divorce, because for a while the logistics just didn't make sense.

At the time I was working the overnight shift and trying to sleep from roughly 5:00 A.M. to noon on weekends, but my husband would wake up at 9:00 A.M. and inevitably wake me up no matter how quiet and careful he tried to be. Because of my insomnia and circadian rhythm, I usually couldn't fall back asleep. I'd be exhausted and cranky the rest of the day, secretly resenting him . . . for opening the door. It got to a point where I'd be getting in bed and already worrying about him waking me up, which of course made it harder for me to sleep. If he dared to make any other noise or movement while I was in bed, I would feel completely exasperated, as if the world was conspiring in some evil plot to keep me from ever sleeping again (remember, insomniacs are prone to catastrophic thinking).

It's easy to understand how this can foster a lot of frustration and resentment, and why moving to another room can be a quick fix that actually improves your relationship.

Dan says for him and Bianca, sleeping in separate rooms "definitely reduced frustration with one another, and boosted our respective sleep quotient. So I would have to say it's been quite positive."

But it's not lost on me that many don't have the luxury of a spare room. In fact, now that we have a child, I no longer do. The good news is, while a sleep divorce can be helpful it's not a necessity. For me, since addressing my insomnia through some of the methods in part 2 of this book and my circadian rhythm issues through some of the methods in part 3 of this book, falling asleep comes much more easily. That means on the rare occasion my husband does wake me up, I no longer get angry or anxious, I just roll over and go back to sleep . . . and because I'm not angry or anxious, I do fall asleep. Also thanks to the tools above and my improved sleep quality from the other tools in this book, those wake-ups rarely happen anymore anyway.

EPILOGUE

It's been a long road for me, from disregarding sleep, to being desperate for sleep, to obsessively learning about sleep, to eventually fixing my sleep—and my husband, Tom, has been a witness to it all.

When we started dating, I was at the Fox Business Network, trying to adjust to my new 3:00 A.M. wake-up time. From there I went to CBS New York, where to my surprise I was quickly thrust into an even earlier schedule. Finally, I came to ABC News, where what started as an overnight shift turned into an overnight plus "whenever anyone possibly asks if I'm available" shift.

Since I'm naturally very energetic, especially in the evening, and Tom's a little more subdued, especially in the evening, he used to joke that the only reason we worked so well as a couple was that I was always slightly sleep-deprived. Even with my early hours I was usually the one trying to convince him, and everyone else, to stay out "just a little bit longer." "Imagine if she were operating at 100 percent," he'd often say. "She'd break me!" Our friends would laugh and nod in agreement. Little did we know, as the years went on, I would end up being the broken one.

As Tom proudly watched my career unfold, he simultaneously watched my sleep problems unfold with it. A mild circadian rhythm disorder became a severe circadian rhythm disorder, which brought on mild insomnia and eventually severe insomnia. But while I thought these issues were inevitable because of my hours, I didn't realize, until recently, that Tom thought these issues were inevitable—because of me.

We were sitting on our couch talking about this book when he suddenly blurted out, "I just can't believe it's not a thing anymore!"

I was confused. "What's not a thing anymore?" I asked.

"You, not sleeping! I always thought your sleep issues were ge-netic or intrinsic to your character and that's just how you would al-ways be. I thought your sleep was fundamentally broken. And now it's just not a thing anymore!" The relief in his voice was palpable, which was surprising to me, not because of the sentiment itself, but because he was feeling it *now*. It had been almost three years since I fixed my sleep problems.

But as I reflected more, I realized that my newfound knowledge about the science of sleep has made my recovery feel more solid. I still have factors that predispose me to insomnia, and Tom wasn't wrong, I likely inherited most, if not all, of them from my parents. But I know now that I have the ability to sleep well despite that.

More importantly, in searching for my sleep fix I haven't just learned a bunch of tools that work for *now*. I've acquired a broad understanding of how and why they work and which ones work best for me. That means I can keep adjusting these tools as the cir-cumstances of my life inevitably change.

It's that understanding that makes me wish there were a few things I could have told myself from the beginning:

1. Attitude Is Everything

I know I've written about having a relaxed or passive attitude a lot throughout this book, but that's only because I think it is the least obvious, most typically ignored, and most crucial piece to this whole puzzle. Virtually no sleep tool will work if we anxiously mon-itor its results, especially if you're an insomniac. If you find yourself thinking, *Okay, I did* [fill in the blank], *NOW let's see if I sleep!* the answer will almost always be no.

Instead, recovering from insomnia is kind of like looking at a 3D Magic Eye picture. Our first instinct is to focus really hard, stare at every part of the picture, and then get frustrated. Inevitably some jerk comes along and sees it right away, which makes us even more frustrated. We try to focus even harder, we try squinting, we want so badly to see this stupid picture! But for all our effort—nothing. Then at some point, we almost give up. We keep looking at the picture, but we stop trying. We zone out and stop thinking about the picture at all, and as we relax our focus, to our surprise, suddenly there it is! A sailboat!

In the same way when you have trouble sleeping, sleep may feel elusive, and it's completely normal to try to fix the problem by sheer force of will and effort. But often it's when we learn to stop trying so hard and stop focusing so much on our sleep, that sleep finally comes. Because sleep is not something we do, sleep is something that happens to us.

2. Set the Table

Having a relaxed attitude can sound a lot like "do nothing" or "give up," but these are not the same thing. Every time I try to reconcile these points, I feel like Paul Rudd in *Forgetting Sarah Marshall,* giving the hilarious surfing instructions: "Don't do anything" and "No, you gotta do more than that!" Not exactly helpful, I realize.

Instead, think of sleep more like a dinner party. You don't want to force-feed your guests or stare at them to carefully monitor their eating. But if you want them to sit and eat with you, you do still want to prepare the food, set the table, and otherwise create an inviting environment.

Same with the 3D picture. To see the image, our focus has to be relaxed, *but* our eyes still have to be open, we still have to be looking at the picture, the lights have to be on, etc.

When it comes to sleep, we don't want to put too much pressure on ourselves, but we still want to foster a good opportunity for sleep to arrive. That's what this book aims to do: to help you create a sleep-friendly scenario, by lowering arousal, limiting outside or internal disruptions, and harnessing the power of your sleep drive and circadian rhythm—in whatever ways make the most sense for you.

But after that, your work is done. You've extended the invitation, and as Dorinda Medley would say, you "made it nice." Now it's up to sleep to join you or not, and it's up to you to try to enjoy yourself regardless. The more relaxed you are, the more likely sleep is to show up, and the more often sleep shows up, the more relaxed you become.

3. Find the Difference Maker

A book's worth of sleep tools can seem overwhelming, so as I said in the beginning, it's important to remember that you don't have to do it all and you definitely don't have to do it all at once.

Instead, if chapter 1 leads you to suspect you have a disorder like sleep apnea, narcolepsy, or RLS, start by addressing that. Otherwise, ask yourself two questions:

1. Do I have conditioned arousal (chapter 3)?
   YES: Try the tools in chapters 3 through 5.
   NO: Move on to question 2.

2. What's different now vs. when I slept well?

If, for example, your caffeine habits have changed since your sleep problems started, you may want to address that. But if you've always had coffee in the afternoon and it never bothered you before, removing that afternoon cup is unlikely to resolve your sleep problem. And without big results, all the sacrifice you make to give up that cup of coffee is probably just going to leave you frustrated. This will arguably have a more negative impact on your sleep than the caffeine did. So leave the coffee alone for now. Once you've resolved the bigger issues disrupting your sleep, you can then try cutting back on caffeine as a way of improving sleep even further.

On the other hand, my answer to question 2 was that I slept well when I had a later work schedule and could go to bed and wake up late. I also slept better on weekends, again, when I could sleep later. Since I couldn't change my work schedule, the next best thing was to adjust my light exposure. So in addition to addressing my conditioned arousal with the tools in part 2 of this book, I also used the tools in chapters 8 and 22 as a starting point. Because these were my difference makers, addressing them had a big impact on my sleep in just a few short weeks. Not only did that motivate me to try other changes, but it gave me a huge boost in my sleep confidence, which generated its own sleep gains.

Find your difference makers and go from there.

4. Done Is Better Than Perfect

As a perfectionist, I need this reminder in almost all aspects of my life—but it's especially important when it comes to sleep advice. Because it's unrealistic to expect everyone to be able to implement every sleep solution exactly as written.

So use the explanations in this book to figure out how to adjust these tools to fit into your life, while still maintaining the same general spirit of what they're trying to accomplish. Don't obsess too much over the details and don't conclude that because you can't do something perfectly, it's not worth doing at all. In the words of Dr. Michael Grandner, "No one is judging you on your form."

5. The Snowball Rolls Both Ways

The most annoying part about sleep trouble is so much of it is like a snowball effect. Sleep is such a crucial pillar in our health that the solution to so many problems is: get more sleep. But when sleep *is* the problem, it makes you feel like the boy in the kid's song "There's a Hole in My Bucket," who's told in order to fix his bucket, he'll need . . . a bucket. "Why can't I sleep? You're too stressed. How do I reduce my stress? Get more sleep!" "How do I improve my sleep? Stop eating at night. Why do I crave food at night? Because you don't sleep enough!" It's hard to not feel hopeless and incredibly lonely. Because no one else seems to get it.

But when we find the difference makers, set the table, and then get out of the way, we realize the beautiful thing about that snowball effect: it also works in the other direction.

This is why, in addition to not having to do it all at once or do it all perfectly, you also don't have to do it all forever.

I, for example, still find that loose stimulus control rules (chapter 5), a really dark room, a light snack before bed if I feel hungry, temperature control tools, and some kind of sound masking help ensure I almost always get a good night's sleep. I will probably do these forever.

But there are many tools that helped me in the beginning that I no longer need.

Some things just become ingrained, like constructive worry (chapter 3). Dr. Nick Wignall says after two to three weeks of doing it daily, most of his patients find their brain just starts doing it automatically, as was my case. From there, you no longer need to do the actual writing exercise every day. You can just save it for when you're feeling stressed.

Some things become easier, like in my case, my diet. As my sleep improved, I found I had fewer cravings for unhealthy food and fewer overnight cravings in general. So after a short while it didn't involve much sacrifice to have healthier, better-timed meals. This was a problem that almost resolved itself.

And finally, some things become less necessary. Looking at my phone used to really stimulate me before bed. But now that my arousal levels are lower and my sleep is better, I find I can mess around on my phone for a bit (in dark and grayscale modes, with the screen extra dim and the color tone warmed) and I still fall asleep just fine. And despite my realization that things like temperature control and sound masking *help* my sleep, I no longer *need* them to sleep and I don't need them to be perfect. I do still need a really dark environment or a sleep mask, but just give me a room that's a reasonable temperature and is fairly quiet and I'm usually fine.

With the 3D picture, the more you do it, the more natural that feeling of relaxing your focus becomes and the better you get at it. Soon you're the jerk who can see the sailboat immediately! It's the same with sleep. Better sleep begets better sleep.

6. Feeling > Hours

Notice I said better sleep begets better sleep—not necessarily more sleep. It's not about how many hours you get. It's about how you feel. If you get six hours of sleep but feel fine during the day, that's probably enough for you. On the other hand, if you get eight hours of sleep but constantly feel like you need a nap, something is wrong.

And no matter how many hours you get or how sleepy you are, if after trying the tools in this book you're still worried about your sleep, contact a professional. Sleep problems are not something anyone should just have to live with, and professional help can change your life or even save your life.

Back on our couch, I gazed back at Tom, so grateful that resolving my sleep problems not only improved my life but clearly made his better too.

But I was still trying to put my finger on why he was so surprised that I could actually be a healthy sleeper when it dawned on me: in our eight years together, he's never known me without sleep problems until now.

"So, what do you think?" I responded, my arms out, inviting his appraisal.

"Thank God we now have a kid to exhaust you, or you would still totally break me."

ACKNOWLEDGMENTS

THERE ARE SO MANY PEOPLE who made *The Sleep Fix* possible.

First and foremost, my husband, Tom. Thank you for always supporting me and my career, even when it meant I had to live like a vampire; for all the tiptoeing you did around me, both literally and figuratively, during my horrible struggle with insomnia; for the many hours of solo parenting you did so that I could write this thing; and for the countless hours you spent reading my drafts, being my analogy tester, and giving me endless amounts of helpful feedback—never once complaining that you were tired of talking about sleep. For that and so much more, I love you.

Fu, after twenty years of friendship you still never cease to amaze me. From bouncer, to DJ, to partner in crime, to man of honor, to Uncle Fu. You can now add "book consultant" to the long list of vital roles you've played in my life. Thank you for always making time for me no matter how busy you are, for still helping me to make decisions I should be able to make on my own, and for always having the right answers—because you're not only insanely smart, you're also incredibly thoughtful. You're the best friend a girl could ask for and this is just one more reason I'm forever indebted to you.

Refet, thank you for the constant generosity of your time and honesty. I can always count on you to give it to me straight and push me to aim higher. As a result, this book and I are both so much better for it.

Thank you to Dr. Michael Breus, Dr. Timothy Brown, Dr. Helen Burgess, Dr. Colleen Carney, Dr. Thomas Dickson, Dr. Christopher Drake, Cara Dumaplin, Dr. Charmane Eastman, Dr. Jason Ellis,

Dr. Daniel Erichsen, Dr. Mariana Figueiro, Dr. Michael Grandner, Dr. Jonathan Johnston, Eliza Kane, Corinne Lederhouse, Nick Littlehales, Dr. Steven Lockley, Dr. Jennifer Mundt, Dr. John O'Neill, Dr. Jason Ong, Dr. Satchin Panda, Dr. Christina Pierpaoli Parker, Dr. Rahbar Rahimpour, Dr. Roy Raymann, Dr. Carolin Reichert, Dr. Timothy Roehrs, Dr. Till Roenneberg, Dr. Clifford Saper, Carolyn Schur, Dr. Hannah Scott, Heather Darwall-Smith, Dr. Jordan Stern, Dr. Marie-Pierre St-Onge, Dr. Joseph Takahashi, Dr. S. Justin Thomas, Dr. Annie Vallières, Dr. Ryan Vandrey, Dr. Janine Weibel, Dr. Nick Wignall, Dr. Chris Winter, Dr. Ken Wright, Dr. Jade Wu, Dr. James Wyatt, Dr. Paul Young, Dr. Shawn Youngstedt, and all the other #SleepPeeps who helped me in ways big and small. When I first started reaching out to you all, I expected to be shut out. I felt a bit like someone asking a magician to reveal how they do their tricks, and expected that you would want to protect the information you worked so hard to learn. Instead I was greeted with support and enthusiasm as I tried to piece together this giant sleep puzzle. Some of you have spent hours on the phone with me; answered countless emails, texts, and tweets; and still found the time to provide me with extra words of encouragement, repeatedly telling me, "You're going to help so many people!" Thank you for welcoming me and trusting me.

To Kofi Kingston, Jason Karp, Janine Elliot, Liz Sobel, Andrea Grymes, Jack Sheahan, Trevor Ault, Eva Pilgrim, Ginger Zee, Adam Amdur, Kevin Freeman, Rosa, and Brad, thank you for sharing your stories with me—they made this book come to life. Special shoutout to Dan Harris, who, despite being one of the busiest people I know, was so generous with his time to encourage me to write this book, teach me what to do to make it happen, and offer so much helpful advice along the way—including changing the title.

To my forever work husband, Kendis Gibson. Not only did you share your sleep story with me, but you were by my side through a large portion of my own sleep journey. Thank you for bringing so much joy to an otherwise difficult time in my life, and for all the other ways you have been and continue to be there for me. On that note, thank you to Bryan Keinz, Briana Stewart, Kim Randolph, Donna Soto, Tinayn Mahler, Jamina Lawrence, Katia Doumbia, Will Ganss, Donna Schroeder, Sandy Panfel, Elena Genovese-Picard, Kris Campbell, Lourdes Leahy, Ronnie Reiss, Matt Nelko, Tony Muzyka, Cristian Roscher, Gentrix Shanga, George Pilla, Debbie Humes, Carla Brittain, Lloyd De Vries, Constance Johnson, Craig Morancie, Noel Lane, Mark Dicso, Joshua Hoyos, Rachel Katz, Matt Foster, and everyone else on the overnight crew at ABC News. I'm still so appreciative of the time I got to spend with all of you and the magic moments we created. Looking back I also know there were times I must have been legitimately crazy due to insomnia and sleep deprivation, so my apologies for anytime I was moody, cranky, or otherwise insane. Special thanks to Greig Todd and Ken Kneeland for allowing and encouraging me to go on this sleep fixing mission for not only my own benefit but for our viewers as well. Were it not for that I may never have set out on this journey at all.

Thanks to Lisa Sharkey, Anna Montague, Tavia Kowalchuk, Christina Joell, and everyone else at HarperCollins who worked on this book, as well as my literary agent, Mel Berger; you decided to take on this project when it was nothing but a vision. Thank you for believing in that vision, for believing in me to bring it to life, and for helping me every step of the way. I also can't forget my TV agent, Ken Lindner, who was not only one of the first people to encourage me to write this book but, as with every other aspect of my career, played such an instrumental role in making it a reality. Thank you for always being my number-one cheerleader. I truly don't know where I'd be without you.

Ryanto, thank you for taking my bizarre visions for sleepy stick figures and making them even better than I imagined. To Bob Kirsch, thank you for saving me from a complete bibliography-induced meltdown. And, Bill Patrick, thank you for your kindness and integrity.

To my bosses and colleagues at ABC, including Kimberly Brown, Derek Medina, Galen Gordon, Mary Noonan, Justin Dial, Wendy Fisher, James Goldston, Michael Kreisel, David Reiter, Dr. Jennifer Ashton, Robin Roberts, Michael Strahan, George Stephanopoulos, David Muir, Amy Robach, Juju Chang, Byron Pitts, TJ Holmes, Linsey Davis, Deborah Roberts, Erielle Reshef, Janai Norman, Gio Benitez, Will Reeve, Rebecca Jarvis, Kenneth Moton, Maggie Rulli, James Longman, Simone Swink, Alberto Orso, Vanessa Webber, Monica Escobedo, Tony Morrison, Eric Jones, Cleopatra Andreadis, Taylor Rhodes, Amy Hayden, and so many more, thank you for your various contributions to a job that I love so much and for supporting me as I pursued this passion project along the way (and occasionally babysitting during live shots). Special shoutout to Katie Dendaas, David Hatcher, Cat McKenzie, Seni Tienabeso, Terry Moran, Molly Shaker, Josh Ascher, Cait Fallon, Matt Claiborne, Megan Hughes, Heidi Jensen, Melissa Kasiarz, Christopher Lumsden, Kyle Mckenzie, Olga Delauz, Olivia Fasano, Rachel Hein, David Merrell, Amari Mitchell, Gabe Rivera, DJ Cunningham, Kelly Carrion, Joselyn Castro, Davi Merchan, Jim Vojtech, Danielle Peake, Sheila Edwards, Flavio Jawor, Rafael Jimenez, Paul Falcone, Dante Dottin, Lisa Christon, and the rest of the ABC News Live "fam." And special thank-you to Curt Villarosa for all your hard work in helping to promote this book.

The Sleep Junkies podcast team, listening to your podcast was some of my favorite kind of research and offered a lot of inspiration throughout my process of writing this book.

Diana, Eileen, Rose, Whitney, and Victoria, thank you for being my tribe and always being there for decisions big and small. My book cover, my wardrobe choices, and my life in general would not be the same without you.

To my family both by blood and by marriage. I won't name you all—both for privacy reasons and because there are way too many of you—but you have done so much for me throughout my life all the way down to covering the windows with garbage bags to try to help me sleep. I couldn't ask for a better support system. Thank you for teaching and showing me what real love is. And a special shout-out to my parents. My work ethic, my values, almost everything that makes me me comes from you and the many lessons you've taught me. Your sleep problems, along with my own, inspired me to write this book, but you have both been an inspiration to me far beyond that. Thank you doesn't cover it.

I hope I've made you all proud—and I hope I've helped you sleep!

NOTES

Chapter 1: Identifying the Problem

11 don't seek professional help: T. Roth and S. Ancoli-Israel, "Daytime consequences and correlates of insomnia in the United States: Results of the 1991 National Sleep Foundation Survey. II." *Sleep* 22, suppl. 2 (1999): S354–S358.

13 circadian rhythm disorder: Erin E. Flynn-Evans, Julia A. Shekleton, Belinda Miller, et al. "Circadian phase and phase angle disorders in primary insomnia." *Sleep* 40, no. 12 (2017): zsx163.

16 thirty and sixty-nine years old: Adam V. Benjafield, Najib T. Ayas, Peter R. Eastwood, et al. "Estimation of the global prevalence and burden of obstructive sleep apnoea: A literature-based analysis." *The Lancet: Respiratory Medicine* 7, no. 8 (2019): P687–P698.

17 other sleep disordered breathing: Vernon D. Rowe, Kenneth R. Van-Owen, John A. Hunter, and Travis Mecum, "Insomnia May Be More of a Breathing Disorder Than Previously Thought," Rowe Neurology Institute, accessed March 3, 2021, www.neurokc.com/wp-content/uploads/2014/09/4-x-4-Poster-Insomnia-May-Be-More-of-a-Breathing-Disorder-than-Previously-Thought.pdf; Sree Roy, "A missing link: Dr. Barry Krakow's research on insomnia and SDB." *Sleep Review*, January 22, 2014, www.sleepreviewmag.com/2014/01/a-missing-link-dr-barry-krakow-s-research-on-insomnia-and-sdb/.

17 compared to white Americans: Abhinav Singh and Logan Foley, "What's the Connection Between Race and Sleep Disorders?" Sleep Foundation, updated July 30, 2020, https://www.sleepfoundation.org/how-sleep-works/whats-connection-between-race-and-sleep-disorders; Katherine A. Dudley and Sanjay R. Patel, "Disparities and genetic risk factors in obstructive sleep apnea." *Sleep Medicine* 18 (2016): 96–102.

17 "untreated sleep apnea": Dayna A. Johnson, Chandra L. Jackson, Natasha J. Williams, and Carmela Alcántara, "Are sleep patterns influenced by race/ethnicity–a marker of relative advantage or disadvantage? Evidence to date." *Nature and Science of Sleep* 11 (2019): 79–95.

18 restless legs, anxiety, and depression: Alison Wimms, Holger Woehrle, Sahisha Ketheeswaran, et al., "Obstructive sleep apnea in women: Specific issues and interventions." *BioMed Research International* 2016 (2016): 1764837; Michael J. Breus, "New Findings on Sleep Apnea in Women," Psychology Today Sleep Newzzz, June 26, 2019, www.psychologytoday.com/us/blog/sleep-newzzz/201906/new-findings-sleep-apnea-in-women.

19 90 percent go undiagnosed: Nathan Alexander, Ahmad Boota, Kenderic Hooks, and John R. White, "Rapid maxillary expansion and adenotonsillectomy in 9-year-old twins with pediatric obstructive sleep apnea syndrome: An interdisciplinary effort." *Journal of the American Osteopathic Association* 119, no. 2 (2019): 126–34.

21   might be at higher risk: American Osteopathic Association, "Researchers
      Say Up to 15% of Children Have Sleep Apnea, Yet 90% Go Undiagnosed,"
      February 12, 2019, www.prnewswire.com/news-releases/researchers-say-up-to
      -15-of-children-have-sleep-apnea-yet-90-go-undiagnosed-300793538.html.

21   diagnosis of sleep apnea: Amir Bar, Giora Pillar, Itsik Dvir, et al. "Eval-
      uation of a portable device based on peripheral arterial tone for unattended
      home sleep studies." *Chest* 123, no. 3 (2003): 695–703; Rafael Golpe, Antonio
      Jiménez, and Rosario Carpizo, "Home sleep studies in the assessment of sleep
      apnea/hypopnea syndrome." *Chest* 122, no. 4 (2002): 1156–61.

21   CPAP long term: Brian W. Rotenberg, Dorian Murariu, and Kenny P.
      Pang, "Trends in CPAP adherence over twenty years of data collection: A
      flattened curve." *Journal of Otolaryngology—Head & Neck Surgery* 45, no. 1
      (2016): 1–9.

23   "the RLS symptoms": Johns Hopkins Medicine. "Causes of Restless
      Legs Syndrome," https://www.hopkinsmedicine.org/neurology_neurosurgery
      /centers_clinics/restless-legs-syndrome/what-is-rls/causes.html.

23   reduce symptoms of rest leg syndrome: Magdolna Hornyak, Ulrich
      Voderholzer, Fritz Hohagen, et al., "Magnesium therapy for periodic leg
      movements—related insomnia and restless legs syndrome: An open pilot
      study." *Sleep* 21, no. 5 (1998): 501–5; Sharon Bartell and Sarah Zallek, "Intra-
      venous magnesium sulfate may relieve restless legs syndrome in pregnancy."
      Journal of Clinical Sleep Medicine 2, no. 2 (2006): 187–88.

24   periodic limb movement disorder: Hornyak, Voderholzer, and Hohagen,
      et al. "Magnesium therapy for periodic leg movements-related insomnia and
      restless legs syndrome: An open pilot study"; Bartell and Zallek. "Intravenous
      magnesium sulfate may relieve restless legs syndrome in pregnancy."

25   or sleep paralysis: National Institute of Neurological Disorders and
      Stroke, Narcolepsy Fact Sheet, www.ninds.nih.gov/Disorders/Patient-Care
      giver-Education/Fact-Sheets/Narcolepsy-Fact-Sheet.

26   other disorders listed above: National Institute of Neurological Disorders
      and Stroke, Narcolepsy Fact Sheet.

27   their quality of life: Anoop K. Gupta, Swapnajeet Sahoo, and Sandeep
      Grover, "Narcolepsy in adolescence—a missed diagnosis: A case report." *Inno-
      vations in Clinical Neuroscience* 14, no. 7–8 (2017): 20–23.

27   usually does work: Treating sleep issues often helps improve mental
      health issues, as demonstrated by Peter L. Franzen and Daniel J. Buysse,
      "Sleep disturbances and depression: Risk relationships for subsequent depres-
      sion and therapeutic implications." *Dialogues in Clinical Neuroscience* 10, no. 4
      (2008): 473–81; Kurshid A. Khurshid, "Comorbid insomnia and psychiatric
      disorders: An update." *Innovations in Clinical Neuroscience* 15, no. 3–4 (2018):
      28–32; Vyga Kaufmann, "Understanding 'How Do I Sleep Better,'" Octo-
      ber 22, 2015, www.youtube.com/watch?v=WNj1Y11t_x8; Harvard Mental
      Health Letter, "Sleep and Mental Health: Sleep Deprivation Can Affect Your
      Mental Health," updated March 18, 2019, www.health.harvard.edu/newslet
      ter_article/sleep-and-mental-health.

28 quit any of these: Henry Ford Health System Staff, "The Link Be-
tween Sleep and Nicotine." Henry Ford LiveWell. Henry Ford Health
System, March 28, 2018, www.henryford.com/blog/2018/03/connection-be
tween-sleep-nicotine; Alan J. Budney, Brent A. Moore, Ryan G. Vandrey, and
John R. Hughes, "The time course and significance of cannabis withdrawal."
Journal of Abnormal Psychology 112, no. 3 (2003): 393–402; Alan J. Budney,
John R. Hughes, Brent A. Moore, and Ryan Vandrey, "Review of the validity
and significance of cannabis withdrawal syndrome." *American Journal of Psy-
chiatry* 161, no. 11 (2004): 1967–77.

30 questions deemed optional: Colleen E. Carney, Daniel J. Buysse, Sonia
Ancoli-Israel, et al., "The consensus sleep diary: Standardizing prospective
sleep self-monitoring." *Sleep* 35, no. 2 (2012): 287–302.

34 "identify suspicious events": SnoreLab, "About SnoreLab," www.snorelab
.com/faqs/.

36 just three questions: Harvard Medical School, Division of Sleep Medicine, "Narcolepsy. Self-Evaluation," dev.healthysleep.med.harvard.edu/narco
lepsy/diagnosing-narcolepsy/narcolepsy-self-evaluation.

38 the Gotcha Alarm: Jason Ellis, *The One-Week Insomnia Cure: Learn to
Solve Your Sleep Problems* (London: Ebury Publishing, 2017), unpaginated.
Kindle.

Chapter 2: Insomnia 101

41 high as 60 percent: Swapna Bhaskar, D. Hemavathy, and Shankar Prasad,
"Prevalence of chronic insomnia in adult patients and its correlation with
medical comorbidities." *Journal of Family Medicine and Primary Care* 5, no. 4
(2016): 780–84.

44 remission within a month: Jason G. Ellis, Toby Cushing, and Anne
Germain, "Treating acute insomnia: A randomized controlled trial of a
'single-shot' of cognitive behavioral therapy for insomnia." *Sleep* 38, no. 6
(2015): 971–78.

44 month of early intervention: Charlotte Randall, Sara Nowakowski, and
Jason G. Ellis, "Managing acute insomnia in prison: Evaluation of a 'one-shot'
cognitive behavioral therapy for insomnia (CBT-I) intervention." *Behavioral
Sleep Medicine* 17, no. 6 (2018): 827–36.

46 "formal education directed at sleep": Harvard Medical School, Division
of Sleep Medicine, Medical Education, sleep.hms.harvard.edu/education-train
ing/medical-education.

52 can still be effective: Annemarie I. Luik, Simon D. Kyle, and Colin A.
Espie, "Digital cognitive behavioral therapy (dCBT) for insomnia:
A state-of-the-science review." *Current Sleep Medicine Reports* 3, no. 2 (2017):
48–56.

54 "on CBT techniques": Mayo Foundation for Health Education, "Insomnia treatment: Cognitive behavioral therapy instead of sleeping pills," www
.mayoclinic.org/diseases-conditions/insomnia/in-depth/insomnia-treatment
/art-20046677.

Part 2: Sleep Drive vs. Arousal

57   inviting to a party: Nga Tran, "The Sleep Paradox—How Working
     Harder on Your Sleep Makes It Worse," Brisbane ACT Centre Clinical Psy-
     chology, www.brisbaneactcentre.com.au/sleep-paradox-working-harder-sleep
     -makes-worse/.

Chapter 3: Overactive Mind

64   "reasoning and logic": Jason Ellis, *The One-Week Insomnia Cure: Learn
     to Solve Your Sleep Problems* (London: Ebury Publishing, 2017), unpaginated.
     Kindle.

64   dilate to take in more light: Ivan Vargas, Anna M. Nguyen, Alexandria
     Muench, et al., "Acute and chronic insomnia: What has time and/or hyper-
     arousal got to do with it?" *Brain Sciences* 10, no. 2 (2020): 71.

64   boredom generally facilitates sleep: Allison C. Cooper, "There's a
     Scientific Reason You Can't Stay Awake in Boring Meetings—Here's Why."
     Updated August 11, 2020, www.thehealthy.com/sleep/why-we-fall-asleep
     -when-bored/.

66   a new one begins: Nilong Vyas and Eric Suni, "Stages of Sleep," Sleep
     Foundation, www.sleepfoundation.org/articles/stages-of-sleep.

Chapter 4: Sleep Confidence and Misperception

77   well over an hour: Matt T. Bianchi, Kathryn L. Williams, Scott McKinney,
     and Jeffrey M. Ellenbogen, "The subjective–objective mismatch in sleep percep-
     tion among those with insomnia and sleep apnea." *Journal of Sleep Research* 22,
     no. 5 (2013): 557–68; Mauro Manconi, Raffaele Ferri, Carolina Sagrada, et al.,
     "Measuring the error in sleep estimation in normal subjects and in patients with
     insomnia." *Journal of Sleep Research* 19, no. 3 (2010): 478–86.

Chapter 5: Not Sleepy Enough

86   "pool of blood": Arianna Huffington, *The Sleep Revolution: Transforming
     Your Life, One Night at a Time* (New York: Harmony Books, 2017), 3. Kindle.

87   "may be appropriate": "How Much Sleep Do You Really Need?" National
     Sleep Foundation, October 1, 2020, www.thensf.org/how-many-hours-of
     -sleep-do-you-really-need/.

87   four to six hours: Arisa Hirano, Pei-Ken Hsu, Luoying Zhang, et al.,
     "DEC2 modulates orexin expression and regulates sleep." *Proceedings of the
     National Academy of Sciences* 115, no. 13 (2018): 3434–39; Guangsen Shi, Li-
     juan Xing, David Wu, et al., "A rare mutation of ß1-adrenergic receptor affects
     sleep/wake behaviors." *Neuron* 103, no. 6 (2019): 1044–1055.e.7; National Li-
     brary of Medicine, "Investigating Genetics of Human Natural Short Sleepers."
     www.ncbi.nlm.nih.gov/projects/gap/cgi-bin/study.cgi?study_id=phs001270
     .v1.p1. *Citation note*: The National Library of Medicine study is not a peer-
     reviewed study but was done as a report for a grant.

93   largely maintained after six months: Leon Lack, Hannah Scott, Gorica
     Micic, and Nicole Lovato, "Intensive sleep re-training: From bench to bed-
     side." *Brain Sciences* 7, no. 4 (2017): 33.

94 sleep onset: Hannah Scott, Andrew Mair, Nicole Lovato, and Leon Lack, "Administering intensive sleep retraining to treat chronic insomnia using the Sleep On Cue smartphone application." *Sleep Medicine* 64 (2019): S340.

96 common CBT-I technique: Richard R. Bootzin and Michael L. Perlis, chapter 2, "Stimulus Control Therapy," in Perelman School of Medicine, University of Pennsylvania, *BSM Treatment Protocols for Insomnia*, www.med .upenn.edu/cbti/assets/user-content/documents/btsd—stimuluscontrol-bsmtx protocols.pdf. Note from author: Guidance is loosely based on chapter, as well as other sources in sleep literature.

98 self-help tool as well: Bruce Rybarczyk, Laurin Mack, Jennifer Huang Harris, and Edward Stepanski, "Testing two types of self-help CBT-I for insomnia in older adults with arthritis or coronary artery disease." *Rehabilitation Psychology* 56, no. 4 (2011): 257–66; Bruce Rybarczyk and Laurin Mack, "Self-help treatments for older adults with primary and comorbid insomnia," in ed. S. R. Pandi-Perumal, J. M. Monti, and A. A. Monjan, *Principles and Practice of Geriatric Sleep Medicine* (New York: Cambridge University Press, 2009): 394.

100 sleep compression didn't get a single mention: Richard R. Bootzin and Michael L. Perlis, chapter 2, "Stimulus Control Therapy," and Arthur J. Spielman, Chien-Ming Yang, and Paul B. Glovinsky, chapter 1, "Sleep Restriction Therapy," in Perelman School of Medicine, University of Pennsylvania, *BSM Treatment Protocols for Insomnia*, www.med.upenn.edu/cbti/assets/user-con tent/documents/btsd—advancedsleeprestriction-spielman.pdf.

104 way to increase adenosine is to exercise: M. Dworak, P. Diel, S. Voss, et al., "Intense exercise increases adenosine concentrations in rat brain: Implications for a homeostatic sleep drive." *Neuroscience* 150, no. 4 (2007): 789–95; Janice M. Marshall, "The roles of adenosine and related substances in exercise hyperaemia." *Journal of Physiology* 583, no. 3 (2007): 835–45; Michael Lazarus, Yo Oishi, Theresa E. Bjorness, and Robert W. Greene, "Gating and the need for sleep: Dissociable effects of adenosine A1 and A2A receptors." *Frontiers in Neuroscience* 13 (2019): 740; Harvard Men's Health Watch, "Refueling Your Energy Levels," October 2018; www.health.harvard .edu/staying-healthy/refueling-your-energy-levels; Dirk J. Duncker and Robert J. Bache, "Regulation of coronary blood flow during exercise." *Physiological Reviews* 88, no. 3 (2008): 1009–86.

Chapter 6: Chronotypes

112 very accurate estimate: Jose Arturo Santisteban, Thomas G. Brown, and Reut Gruber, "Association between the Munich Chronotype Questionnaire and wrist actigraphy." *Sleep Disorders* 2018 (2018): 5646848; Shingo Kitamura, Akiko Hida, Sayaka Aritake, et al., "Validity of the Japanese version of the Munich ChronoType Questionnaire." *Chronobiology International* 31, no. 7 (2014): 845–50; K. S. Jankowski, "Composite Scale of Morningness: Psychometric properties, validity with Munich ChronoType Questionnaire and age/sex differences in Poland." *European Psychiatry* 30, no. 1 (2015): 166–71; Sooyeon Suh, Soo Hyun Kim, Hyera Ryu, et al., "Validation of the

Korean Munich Chronotype Questionnaire." *Sleep and Breathing* 22, no. 3 (2018): 773–79.

Chapter 7: Scheduling

115 Indra Nooyi wakes up at 4:00 A.M.: Abigail Johnson Hess, "10 highly successful people who wake up before 6 a.m.," CNBC Make It, May 17, 2018, www.cnbc.com/2018/05/17/10-highly-successful-people-who-wake-up-before -6-a-m.html.

120 doesn't go to bed until around two A.M.: Alexis Ohanian, as told to Sky-lar Bergl, "Most Productive People: Alexis Ohanian," Fast Company, Work Smart, November 18, 2013, www.fastcompany.com/3021642/most-productive -people-reddit-alexis-ohanian.

120 and sleeps until seven: "Tesla CEO Elon Musk," AutoBild, November 5, 2014, www.youtube.com/watch?v=FE4iFYqi4QU&feature=youtu.be &t=2m21s.

120 more of a morning person.: "Mark Zuckerberg, First Ever Live Q&A on Facebook!" June 14, 2016, www.facebook.com/zuck/videos/vb.4 /10102895343490231/?type=2&theater.

121 wakes up at nine: Rachel Gillett, "18 People Who Prove You Don't Have to Wake Up Incredibly Early to Be Successful," *Business Insider*, June 24, 2017, www.businessinsider.com/successful-people-who-wake-up-late-2017-6#musi cian-philanthropist-and-entrepreneur-pharrell-williams-rolls-out-of-bed-at-9 -am-without-an-alarm-clock-13.

Chapter 8: Light/Dark Contrast

126 enough natural daylight: Satchin Panda, *The Circadian Code: Lose Weight, Supercharge Your Energy, and Transform Your Health from Morning to Midnight* (New York: Rodale Books, 2018), 77. Kindle.

127 most participants experienced that drop around 25 lux: Andrew J. K. Phillips, Parisa Vidafar, Angus C. Burns, et al., "High sensitivity and interin-dividual variability in the response of the human circadian system to evening light." *Proceedings of the National Academy of Sciences of the USA* 116, no. 24 (2019): 12019–24.

128 sunglasses can reduce the amount of light: Panda, *Circadian Code*, 168.

129 best time for daily light exposure: Leon Lack and Helen Wright, chap-ter e39, "The Use of Bright Light in the Treatment of Insomnia," in Perelman School of Medicine, University of Pennsylvania, *BSM Treatment Protocols for Insomnia*, www.med.upenn.edu/cbti/assets/user-content/documents/Lack _BrightLightTreatmentofInsomnia.pdf.

129 "workplaces without windows": Mohamed Boubekri, Ivy N. Cheung, Kathryn J. Reid, et al., "Impact of windows and daylight exposure on overall health and sleep quality of office workers: A case-control pilot study." *Journal of Clinical Sleep Medicine* 10, no. 6 (2014): 603611.

129 lenses become thicker and more yellow with age: Suzanne Hood and Shimon Amir, "The aging clock: Circadian rhythms and later life." *Journal of Clinical Investigation* 127, no. 2 (2017): 437–46.

129 total sleep also increased: In-Young Yoon, Do-Un Jeong, Ki-Bum Kwon, et al., "Bright light exposure at night and light attenuation in the morning improve adaptation of night shift workers." *Sleep* 25, no. 3 (2002): 351–56.

129 bright light therapy as "highly effective": Karen T. Stewart, Benita C. Hayes, and Charmane I. Eastman. "Light treatment for NASA shiftworkers." *Chronobiology International* 12, no. 2 (1995): 141–51.

133 powerful response to yellow light: Joshua W. Mouland, Franck Martial, Alex Watson, et al., "Cones support alignment to an inconsistent world by suppressing mouse circadian responses to the blue colors associated with twilight." *Current Biology* 29, no. 24 (2019): 4260–67.e4.

133 cooler light tones in the evening: Michael Addelman, "Researchers Discover When It's Good to Get the Blues" (press release), University of Manchester, December 16, 2019, www.manchester.ac.uk/discover/news /researchers-discover-when-its-good-to-get-the-blues/.

134 human circadian system: The responses of the experts I spoke with are also supported by David C. Holzman, "What's in a color? The unique human health effects of blue light." *Environmental Health Perspectives* 118, no. 1 (2010): A22–A27; Giulia Zerbini, Thomas Kantermann, and Martha Merrow, "Strategies to decrease social jetlag: Reducing evening blue light advances sleep and melatonin." *European Journal of Neuroscience* 51, no. 12 (2020): 2355–66.

134 red bulbs in night-lights: Satchin Panda, *The Circadian Code: Lose Weight, Supercharge Your Energy, and Transform Your Health from Morning to Midnight* (New York: Rodale Books, 2018), 161–62. Kindle.

135 the chart below: Panda, *The Circadian Code,* 129.

137 dark sunglasses during their commute: Yoon, Jeong, Kwon, et al., "Bright light exposure at night and light attenuation in the morning improve adaptation of night shift workers."

137 sunglasses and blue-blocking glasses: F. O. James, E. Chevrier, and D. B. Boivin, "A light/darkness intervention to improve daytime sleep quality in night shift workers." In *XVIth International Symposium on Night and Shiftwork*, vol. 100 (2003); Mark R. Smith, Louis F. Fogg, and Charmane I. Eastman, "Practical interventions to promote circadian adaptation to permanent night shift work: Study 4." *Journal of Biological Rhythms* 24, no. 2 (2009): 161–72; Alexandre Sasseville, Nathalie Paquet, Jean Sévigny, and Marc Hébert, "Blue blocker glasses impede the capacity of bright light to suppress melatonin production." *Journal of Pineal Research* 41, no. 1 (2006): 73–78.

Chapter 9: The Right Way to Take Melatonin

141 clock-shifting potential: Jonathan S. Emens and Helen J. Burgess, "Effect of light and melatonin and other melatonin receptor agonists on human circadian physiology." *Sleep Medicine Clinics* 10, no. 4 (2015): 435–53.

Chapter 10: Body Temperature

146 elevated core body temperatures: Leon C. Lack, Michael Gradisar, Eus J.W. Van Someren, et al., "The relationship between insomnia and body temperatures." *Sleep Medicine Reviews* 12, no. 4 (2008): 307–17.

146 raising core body temp: Nilong Vyas and Eric Suni, "PMS and Insomnia," Sleep Foundation, updated September 15, 2020, www.sleepfoundation .org/articles/6-sleep-problems-occur-during-your-period-and-what-do-make -them-go-away.

147 advanced core temperature rhythm: Eus J. W. Van Someren, Roy J.E.M. Raymann, Erik J.A. Scherder, et al., "Circadian and age-related modulation of thermoreception and temperature regulation: Mechanisms and functional implications." *Ageing Research Reviews* 1, no. 4 (2002): 721–78.

147 decrease in thermosensitivity: Roy J.E.M. Raymann and Eus J.W. Van Someren, "Diminished capability to recognize the optimal temperature for sleep initiation may contribute to poor sleep in elderly people." *Sleep* 31, no. 9 (2008): 1301–9.

147 relays those timing signals: Ethan D. Buhr, Seung-Hee Yoo, and Joseph S. Takahashi. "Temperature as a universal resetting cue for mammalian circadian oscillators." *Science* 330, no. 6002 (2010): 379–85.

149 time it takes to fall asleep: Shahab Haghayegh, Sepideh Khoshnevis, Michael H. Smolensky, et al., "Before-bedtime passive body heating by warm shower or bath to improve sleep: A systematic review and meta-analysis." *Sleep Medicine Reviews* 46 (2019): 124–35.

149 exercise too close to bedtime: Rachel R. Markwald, Imran Iftikhar, and Shawn D. Youngstedt, "Behavioral strategies, including exercise, for addressing insomnia." *ACSM's Health & Fitness Journal* 22, no. 2 (2018): 23–29.

150 "helps to facilitate sleepiness": Johns Hopkins Medicine, "Exercising for Better Sleep," www.hopkinsmedicine.org/health/wellness-and-prevention /exercising-for-better-sleep.

151 "core body temperature too high for sleep": Satchin Panda, *The Circadian Code: Lose Weight, Supercharge Your Energy, and Transform Your Health from Morning to Midnight* (New York: Rodale Press, 2018), 77. Kindle.

152 melatonin deficiency: D. Weinert and D. G. Gubin, "The circadian body temperature rhythm—Origin and implications for health and well-being." Тюменский медицинский журнал 20, no. 2 (2018). cyberleninka .ru/article/n/the-circadian-body-temperature-rhythm-origin-and-implications -for-health-and-wellbeing/viewer.

152 rebound spike in core body temperature: Timothy Roehrs and Thomas Roth, "Sleep, sleepiness, and alcohol use." *Alcohol Research & Health* 25, no. 2 (2001): 101–9.

Chapter 11: Meal Timing

153 spike in the hormone insulin: Priya Crosby, Ryan Hamnett, Marrit Putker, et al. "Insulin/IGF-1 drives PERIOD synthesis to entrain circadian rhythms with feeding time." *Cell* 177, no. 4 (2019): 896–909.e20.

153 crave fat and sugar: Matthew J. Edlund, "Stress, Eating, and Sleep."

Psychology Today, February 8, 2018, www.psychologytoday.com/za/blog/the
-power-rest/201802/stress-eating-and-sleep.

154 first meal of the day: Shubhroz Gill and Satchidananda Panda. "A smartphone app reveals erratic diurnal eating patterns in humans that can be mod-
ulated for health benefits." *Cell Metabolism* 22, no. 5 (2015): 789–98; Michael
J. Wilkinson, Emily N. C. Manoogian, Adena Zadourian, et al., "Ten-hour
time-restricted eating reduces weight, blood pressure, and atherogenic lipids in
patients with metabolic syndrome." *Cell Metabolism* 31, no. 1 (2020): 92–104.

154 "drinking a glass of water": Satchin Panda, *The Circadian Code: Lose
Weight, Supercharge Your Energy, and Transform Your Health from Morning to
Midnight* (New York: Rodale Books, 2018), 102. Kindle.

154 what helps to lower cortisol? Carbs.: Hoda Soltani, Nancy L. Keim, and
Kevin D. Laugero, "Increasing dietary carbohydrate as part of a healthy whole
food diet intervention dampens eight week changes in salivary cortisol and
cortisol responsiveness." *Nutrients* 11, no. 11 (2019): 2563.

156 "no schedule at all": Panda, *Circadian Code*, 106.

156 last meal of the day: Panda, *Circadian Code*, 41.

156 decrease your eating window: Panda, *Circadian Code*, 108.

157 no milk or sweetener: Panda, *Circadian Code*, 108.

157 back on track as soon as you can: Panda, *Circadian Code*, 99.

157 suddenly start seeing progress again: Panda, *Circadian Code*, 110.

157 "match the food availability": Patrick M. Fuller, Jun Lu, and Clifford B.
Saper, "Differential rescue of light- and food-entrainable circadian rhythms."
Science 320, no. 5879 (2008): 1074–77.

159 jet lag returning home: Norman C. Reynolds Jr. and Robert Montgom-
ery, "Using the Argonne diet in jet lag prevention: Deployment of troops
across nine time zones." *Military Medicine* 167, no. 6 (2002): 451–53.

Chapter 12: When to Work Out

161 the effect of exercise: Shawn D. Youngstedt, Jeffrey A. Elliott, and Daniel
F. Kripke, "Human circadian phase-response curves for exercise." *Journal of
Physiology* 597, no. 8 (2019): 2253–68.

161 advance circadian rhythm: Orfeu M. Buxton, Calvin W. Lee, Mireille
L'Hermite-Balériaux, et al., "Exercise elicits phase shifts and acute alterations
of melatonin that vary with circadian phase." *American Journal of Physiology—
Regulatory, Integrative and Comparative Physiology* 284, no. 3 (2003): R714–
R724.

162 night owl chronotypes: Charmane I. Eastman, Erin K. Hoese, Shawn D.
Youngstedt, and Liwen Liu, "Phase-shifting human circadian rhythms with exercise during the night shift." *Physiology & Behavior* 58, no. 6 (1995): 1287–91.

Chapter 13: Sleep Debt Strategies

165 data doesn't support this: Josiane L. Broussard, Kristen Wroblewski,
Jennifer M. Kilkus, and Esra Tasali, "Two nights of recovery sleep reverses the
effects of short-term sleep restriction on diabetes risk." *Diabetes Care* 39, no. 3
(2016): e40–e41.

165 all of those changes reversed: Karine Spiegel, Rachel Leproult, and Eve Van Cauter, "Impact of sleep debt on metabolic and endocrine function." *The Lancet* 354, no. 9188 (1999): 1435–39.

165 sleep debt-related ailments: Yuki Motomura, Shingo Kitamura, Kyoko Nakazaki, et al., "Recovery from unrecognized sleep loss accumulated in daily life improved mood regulation via prefrontal suppression of amygdala activity." *Frontiers in Neurology* 8 (2017): 306.

168 circadian-related negative effects: Michael Breus, *The Power of When: Discover Your Chronotype—And the Best Time to Eat Lunch, Ask for a Raise, Have Sex, Write a Novel, Take Your Meds, and More* (New York: Little, Brown Spark, 2016), 182. Kindle.

168 "gradually shift your body's clock": Reneé Prince, "Say Goodbye to Sleep Debt," Sleep.org, www.sleep.org/articles/say-goodbye-sleep-debt/.

169 60 to 90 minutes: Reneé Prince, "Say Goodbye to Sleep Debt," Sleep.org, www.sleep.org/articles/say-goodbye-sleep-debt/.

169 sleep more efficiently: Sarah M. Jay, Nicole Lamond, Sally A. Ferguson, et al., "The characteristics of recovery sleep when recovery opportunity is restricted." *Sleep* 30, no. 3 (2007): 353–60; UAMS Health, "Can You Make Up for Lost Sleep?" uamshealth.com/medical-myths/can-you-make-up-for-lost-sleep/.

Chapter 14: The Graveyard Shift

178 compared to control groups: Mark R. Smith, Louis F. Fogg, and Charmane I. Eastman, "A compromise circadian phase position for permanent night work improves mood, fatigue, and performance." *Sleep* 32, no. 11 (2009): 1481–89; Mark R. Smith, Louis F. Fogg, and Charmane I. Eastman, "Practical interventions to promote circadian adaptation to permanent night shift work: Study 4." *Journal of Biological Rhythms* 24, no. 2 (2009): 161–72.

179 "night shifts and on days off": Mark R. Smith and Charmane I. Eastman, "Night shift performance is improved by a compromise circadian phase position: Study 3. Circadian phase after 7 night shifts with an intervening weekend off." *Sleep* 31, no. 12 (2008): 1639–45.

180 improve cognitive performance in shift workers: Katharine Ker, Philip James Edwards, Lambert M. Felix, et al., "Caffeine for the prevention of injuries and errors in shift workers." *Cochrane Database of Systematic Reviews* 5 (2010): CD008508.

180 daytime sleep compared to nighttime sleep: Julie Carrier, Marta Fernandez-Bolanos, Rébecca Robillard, et al., "Effects of caffeine are more marked on daytime recovery sleep than on nocturnal sleep." *Neuropsychopharmacology* 32, no. 4 (2007): 964–72.

180 mild and moderate caffeine users: Paula K. Schweitzer, Angela C. Randazzo, Kara Stone, et al., "Laboratory and field studies of naps and caffeine as practical countermeasures for sleep-wake problems associated with night work." *Sleep* 29, no. 1 (2006): 39–50.

180 benefits of caffeine wore off: Tracy Jill Doty, Christine J. So, Elizabeth M.

Bergman, et al., "Limited efficacy of caffeine and recovery costs during and following 5 days of chronic sleep restriction." *Sleep* 40, no. 12 (2017): zsx171.

181 "adverse effects due to night shift work": Hidemaro Takeyama, Tomohide Kubo, and Toru Itani, "The nighttime nap strategies for improving night shift work in workplace." *Industrial Health* 43, no. 1 (2005): 24–29.

181 including car accidents: Sergio Garbarino, Barbara Mascialino, Maria Antonietta Penco, et al., "Professional shift-work drivers who adopt prophylactic naps can reduce the risk of car accidents during night work." *Sleep* 27, no. 7 (2004): 1295–302.

181 "shorter than that without [a] nap": Hidemaro Takeyama, Tomohide Kubo, and Toru Itani, "The nighttime nap strategies for improving night shift work in workplace." *Industrial Health* 43, no. 1 (2005): 24–29.

181 napping overnight: Sanae Oriyama and Yukiko Miyakoshi, "The effects of nighttime napping on sleep, sleep inertia, and performance during simulated 16 h night work: A pilot study." *Journal of Occupational Health* 60, no. 2 (2017): 172–81.

181 little to no sleep inertia: Sree Roy. "For Night Shift Workers, Sleep Inertia Adds Risk to Naps," *Sleep Review*, December 8, 2014. www.sleepreviewmag.com/uncategorized/night-shift-workers-sleep-inertia-risk-naps/.

183 household knows you're sleeping: American Academy of Sleep Medicine, "Provider Fact Sheet: Circadian Adaptation to Shift Work," j2vjt3dnbra3ps7ll1clb4q2-wpengine.netdna-ssl.com/wp-content/uploads/2019/02/ProviderFS_ShiftChanges_19.pdf.

192 evening shift to day shift: American Academy of Sleep Medicine. "Provider Fact Sheet: Circadian Adaptation to Shift Work."

192 at least one day off: American Academy of Sleep Medicine, "Provider Fact Sheet: Circadian Adaptation to Shift Work."

Chapter 15: Booze and Snooze

197 "alcohol to help them fall asleep": Abhinay Singh and Danielle Pacheco, "Alcohol and Sleep," Sleep Foundation, www.sleepfoundation.org/nutrition/alcohol-and-sleep#:~:text=The%20findings%20are%20as%20follows,decreased%20sleep%20quality%20by%2024%25.

198 prone to snoring and sleep apnea: Abhinav Singh and Danielle Pacheco, "Alcohol and Sleep."

198 cortisol rhythm and melatonin rhythm: Alan M. Rosenwasser, "Alcohol, antidepressants, and circadian rhythms: human and animal models." *Alcohol Research & Health* 25, no. 2 (2001): 126–35.

198 alcohol can also make that worse: National Institute of Neurological Disorders and Stroke, "Restless Legs Syndrome Fact Sheet," www.ninds.nih.gov/Disorders/Patient-Caregiver-Education/Fact-Sheets/Restless-Legs-Syndrome-Fact-Sheet.

200 increasing the alcohol metabolic rate: Arthur I. Cederbaum, "Alcohol metabolism." *Clinics in Liver Disease* 16, no. 4 (2012): 667–85.

202 "weird behaviors reported on sleeping pills": Michael J. Breus, "Ten Things You Can Do to Make Your Sleeping Medication or Sleep Supplements

More Effective," The Sleep Doctor, July 7, 2018, thesleepdoctor.com/2018/07 /07/10-things-you-can-do-to-make-your-sleeping-medication-or-sleep-supple ments-more-effective/.

202 defines moderate drinking as: U.S. Department of Health and Human Services and U.S. Department of Agriculture. *2015–2020 Dietary Guidelines for Americans, 8th ed.,* December 2015. health.gov/our-work/food-nutrition /previous-dietary-guidelines/2015.

203 giving up all alcohol: W. Chris Winter, *The Sleep Solution: Why Your Sleep Is Broken and How to Fix It* (New York: New American Library, 2017), 120. Kindle.

Chapter 16: The Truth About Screens

205 nightly emailing and browsing: Rebecca A. Gallagher, Michael L. Perlis, Subhajit Chakravorty, et al., "Use of mobile electronic devices in bed associated with sleep duration, insomnia, and daytime sleepiness." Second Annual CSCN & Penn Chronobiology Program Joint Collaboration Research Retreat, June 17, 2015, https://www.med.upenn.edu/sleepctr/assets/user-con tent/documents/2015%20Abstracts/Khadeer,%20Gallagher,%20Perlis,%20 Chakravorty,%20et%20al.pdf.

206 the more interactive a device: Michael Gradisar, Amy R. Wolfson, Allison G. Harvey, et al., "The sleep and technology use of Americans: Findings from the National Sleep Foundation's 2011 Sleep in America poll." *Journal of Clinical Sleep Medicine* 9, no. 12 (2013): 1291–99.

212 blue-light-blocking software: Reza Kazemi, Negar Alighanbari, and Zahra Zamanian, "The effects of screen light filtering software on cognitive performance and sleep among night workers." *Health Promotion Perspectives* 9, no. 3 (2019): 233.

212 amber-tinted blue-light-blocking glasses: Ari Shechter, Elijah Wookhyun Kim, Marie-Pierre St-Onge, and Andrew J. Westwood, "Blocking nocturnal blue light for insomnia: A randomized controlled trial." *Journal of Psychiatric Research* 96 (2018): 196–202.

Chapter 17: Caffeine All Wrong

216 function of caffeine is to boost cortisol: William R. Lovallo, Thomas L. Whitsett, Mustafa al'Absi, et al., "Caffeine stimulation of cortisol secretion across the waking hours in relation to caffeine intake levels." *Psychosomatic Medicine* 67, no. 5 (2005): 734–39.

216 "coffee in the morning": Michael Breus, *The Power of When: Discover Your Chronotype—And the Best Time to Eat Lunch, Ask for a Raise, Have Sex, Write a Novel, Take Your Meds, and More* (New York: Little, Brown Spark, 2016), 171. Kindle.

216 sleep inertia: Patricia Tassi and Alain Muzet, "Sleep inertia." *Sleep Medicine Reviews* 4, no. 4 (2000): 341–53.

217 caffeine half-life: Justin Evans, John R. Richards, and Amanda S. Battisti, "Caffeine." In *StatPearls [Internet]* (Treasure Island, FL: StatPearls Publishing, 2021).

218 extends half-life: Jennifer L. Temple, Christophe Bernard, Steven E. Lipshultz, et al., "The safety of ingested caffeine: A comprehensive review." *Frontiers in Psychiatry* 8 (2017): 80.

218 400 milligrams of caffeine: Christopher Drake, Timothy Roehrs, John Shambroom, and Thomas Roth, "Caffeine effects on sleep taken 0, 3, or 6 hours before going to bed." *Journal of Clinical Sleep Medicine* 9, no. 11 (2013): 1195–200.

219 delayed subjects' melatonin rhythms: Tina M. Burke, Rachel R. Markwald, Andrew W. McHill, et al., "Effects of caffeine on the human circadian clock in vivo and in vitro." *Science Translational Medicine* 7, no. 305 (2015): 305ra146.

220 delivery form like caffeine gum: Gary H. Kamimori, Chetan S. Karyekar, Ronald Otterstetter, et al. "The rate of absorption and relative bioavailability of caffeine administered in chewing gum versus capsules to normal healthy volunteers." *International Journal of Pharmaceutics* 234, no. 1–2 (2002): 159–67.

221 power nap before the caffeine: Gary H. Kamimori, Chetan S. Karyekar, Ronald Otterstetter, et al., "The rate of absorption and relative bioavailability of caffeine administered in chewing gum versus capsules to normal healthy volunteers." *International Journal of Pharmaceutics* 234, no. 1–2 (2002): 159–67.

221 performance-enhancing effects of caffeine: American Academy of Sleep Medicine, "Caffeine has little to no benefit after 3 nights of sleep restriction," June 12, 2016, aasm.org/caffeine-has-little-to-no-benefit-after-3-nights-of-sleep-restriction/.

223 "gusto of your digestion": Shawn Stevenson, *Sleep Smarter: 21 Essential Strategies to Sleep Your Way to a Better Body, Better Health, and Bigger Success* (New York: Rodale, 2016), 256. Kindle.

224 "acute" evening caffeine: Janine Weibel, Yu-Shiuan Lin, Hans-Peter Landolt, et al., "Caffeine-dependent changes of sleep-wake regulation: Evidence for adaptation after repeated intake." *Progress in Neuro-Psychopharmacology & Biological Psychiatry* 99 (2020): 109851.

Chapter 18: To Eat or Not to Eat

225 sleeping on an empty stomach: Jennifer Hines, "Why I can't sleep: 6 common reasons and fixes to help you sleep through the night," Alaska Sleep Education Center, May 22, 2018, www.alaskasleep.com/blog/why-i-cant-sleep-6-common-reasons-and-fixes-to-help-you-sleep-thru-the-night.

225 Acid reflux: Rene Wisely, "Why Sleep Disorders Cause Heartburn (and Vice Versa)," Michigan Health, March 13, 2018, healthblog.uofmhealth.org/digestive-health/why-sleep-disorders-cause-heartburn-and-vice-versa.

226 carbs help lower cortisol: Hoda Soltani, Nancy L. Keim, and Kevin D. Laugero, "Increasing dietary carbohydrate as part of a healthy whole food diet intervention dampens eight week changes in salivary cortisol and cortisol responsiveness." *Nutrients* 11, no. 11 (2019): 2563.

226 participants' usual eating habits: Adam Kirstine, "Dietary habits and sleep after bedtime food drinks." *Sleep* 3, no. 1 (1980): 47–58.

227 a lighter pre-bed snack: Marie-Pierre St-Onge, Anja Mikic, and Cara E. Pietrolungo, "Effects of diet on sleep quality." *Advances in Nutrition 7*, no. 5 (2016): 938–49; Wilfred R. Pigeon, Michelle Carr, Colin Gorman, and Michael L. Perlis, "Effects of a tart cherry juice beverage on the sleep of older adults with insomnia: A pilot study." *Journal of Medicinal Food* 13, no. 3 (2010): 579–83; María Garrido, Sergio D. Paredes, Javier Cubero, et al., "Jerte Valley cherry-enriched diets improve nocturnal rest and increase 6-sulfatoxymelatonin and total antioxidant capacity in the urine of middle-aged and elderly humans." *Journals of Gerontology Series A: Biological Sciences and Medical Sciences* 65, no. 9 (2010): 909–14.

Chapter 19: Sleep Nutrition

229 sleep deprivation leads us to eat: Marie-Pierre St-Onge and Faris M. Zuraikat, "Reciprocal roles of sleep and diet in cardiovascular health: A review of recent evidence and a potential mechanism." *Current Atherosclerosis Reports* 21, no. 3 (2019): 11.

230 healthy levels of the neurotransmitter GABA: S. B. Sartori, N. Whittle, A. Hetzenauer, and N. Singewald, "Magnesium deficiency induces anxiety and HPA axis dysregulation: Modulation by therapeutic drug treatment." *Neuropharmacology* 62, no. 1 (2012): 304–12.

230 National Sleep Foundation, "Power (Down) Vitamins: Promote Better Sleep with Magnesium," Sleep.org, www.sleep.org/power-vitamins-promote -better-sleep-magnesium/.

230 reduce cortisol, stress, and anxiety: S. W. Golf, O. Happel, V. Graef, and K. E. Seim, "Plasma aldosterone, cortisol and electrolyte concentrations in physical exercise after magnesium supplementation." *Journal of Clinical Chemistry and Clinical Biochemistry* 22, no. 11 (1984): 717–21; Neil Bernard Boyle, Clare Lawton, and Louise Dye, "The effects of magnesium supplementation on subjective anxiety and stress—a systematic review." *Nutrients* 9, no. 5 (2017): 429; H. Murck, "Magnesium and affective disorders." *Nutritional Neuroscience* 5, no. 6 (2002): 375–89; E. A. Tarasov, D. V. Blinov, U. V. Zimovina, and E. A. Sandakova, "Magnesium deficiency and stress: Issues of their relationship, diagnostic tests, and approaches to therapy." *Therapeutic Archive* 87, no. 9 (2015): 114–22.

230 restless or "broken" sleep: Michael J. Breus, "What You Need to Know About Magnesium and Your Sleep," May 14, 2018, www.psychologytoday .com/us/blog/sleep-newzzz/201805/what-you-need-know-about-magnesium -and-your-sleep.

231 periodic limb movement disorder: Magdolna Hornyak, Ulrich Voderholzer, Fritz Hohagen, et al., "Magnesium therapy for periodic leg movements-related insomnia and restless legs syndrome: An open pilot study." *Sleep* 21, no. 5 (1998): 501–5; Sharon Bartell and Sarah Zallek, "Intravenous magnesium sulfate may relieve restless legs syndrome in pregnancy." *Journal of Clinical Sleep Medicine* 2, no. 2 (2006): 187–88.

231 magnesium deficient: Adela Hruby and Nicola M. McKeown, "Mag-

nesium deficiency: What is our status?" *Nutrition Today* 51, no. 3 (2016): 121–28.

231 more magnesium you need: James J. DiNicolantonio, James H. O'Keefe, and William Wilson, "Subclinical magnesium deficiency: A principal driver of cardiovascular disease and a public health crisis." *Open Heart* 5, no. 1 (2018): e000668.

232 higher dosage of topical magnesium: Uwe Gröber, Tanja Werner, Jürgen Vormann, and Klaus Kisters, "Myth or reality—transdermal magnesium?" *Nutrients* 9, no. 8 (2017): 813; Lindsy Kass, Andrea Rosanoff, Amy Tanner, et al., "Effect of transdermal magnesium cream on serum and urinary magnesium levels in humans: A pilot study." *PloS One* 12, no. 4 (2017): e0174817; Akira Kuriyama, Hirokazu Maeda, and Rao Sun, "Topical application of magnesium to prevent intubation-related sore throat in adult surgical patients: a systematic review and meta-analysis." *Canadian Journal of Anesthesia/Journal canadien d'anesthésie* 66, no. 9 (2019): 1082–94; Ibrahim Al Bakir, Franklin Adaba, Kinesh Patel, and Jeremy Nightingale, "PWE-109 Topical magnesium therapy treats hypomagnesaemia in some ileostomy patients." *Gut* 67, suppl. 1 (2018): A172.2–A173.

232 placebo effect on insomnia: Michael L. Perlis, W. Vaughn McCall, Carla R. Jungquist, et al., "Placebo effects in primary insomnia." *Sleep Medicine Reviews* 9, no. 5 (2005): 381–89.

233 tryptophan has been shown: Trisha A. Jenkins, Jason C.D. Nguyen, Kate E. Polglaze, and Paul P. Bertrand, "Influence of tryptophan and serotonin on mood and cognition with a possible role of the gut-brain axis." *Nutrients* 8, no. 1 (2016): 56.

233 daily intake of tryptophan: Harris R. Lieberman, Sanjiv Agarwal, and Victor L. Fulgoni III, "Tryptophan intake in the US adult population is not related to liver or kidney function but is associated with depression and sleep outcomes." *Journal of Nutrition* 146, no. 12 (2016): 2609S–2615S.

233 many other amino acids: National Sleep Foundation, "What Is Tryptophan?" Sleep.org, www.sleep.org/articles/what-is-tryptophan/.

234 potentially impairing sleep: James E. Gangwisch, Lauren Hale, Marie-Pierre St-Onge, et al., "High glycemic index and glycemic load diets as risk factors for insomnia: Analyses from the Women's Health Initiative." *American Journal of Clinical Nutrition* 111, no. 2 (2020): 429–39; Nilong Vyas and Eric Suni, "The Best Foods to Help You Sleep," Sleep Foundation, www.sleepfoundation.org/articles/food-and-drink-promote-good-nights-sleep.

235 B_6 deficiency: Jennifer Hines, "Food for Sleep: The Best and Worst Foods for Getting Sleep," Alaska Sleep Education Center, www.alaskasleep.com/blog/foods-for-sleep-list-best-worst-foods-getting-sleep-0.

235 11 percent had low levels: Martha Savaria Morris, Mary Frances Picciano, Paul F. Jacques, and Jacob Selhub, "Plasma pyridoxal 5-phosphate in the US population: The National Health and Nutrition Examination Survey, 2003–2004." *American Journal of Clinical Nutrition* 87, no. 5 (2008): 1446–54; National Institutes of Health, Office of Dietary Supplements,

"Vitamin B$_6$: Fact Sheet for Health Professionals," ods.od.nih.gov/factsheets /VitaminB6-HealthProfessional/#en12.

236 remember our dreams: Denholm J. Aspy, Natasha A. Madden, and Paul Delfabbro, "Effects of vitamin B$_6$ (pyridoxine) and a B complex preparation on dreaming and sleep." *Perceptual and Motor Skills* 125, no. 3 (2018): 451–62.

236 sufficient amount of vitamin D: Omeed Sizar, Swapnil Khare, Amandeep Goyal, et al., "Vitamin D deficiency." *StatPearls [Internet]* (Treasure Island, FL: StatPearls Publishing, 2020).

237 the lower the vitamin D levels: Conor P. Kerley, Katrina Hutchinson, Kenneth Bolger, et al., "Serum vitamin D is significantly inversely associated with disease severity in Caucasian adults with obstructive sleep apnea syndrome." *Sleep* 39, no. 2 (2016): 293–300; T. Mete, Y. Yalcin, D. Berker, et al., "Obstructive sleep apnea syndrome and its association with vitamin D deficiency." *Journal of Endocrinological Investigation* 36, no. 9 (2013): 681–85.

237 increased risk of skin cancer: National Institutes of Health, Office of Dietary Supplements, "Vitamin D: Fact Sheet for Health Professionals," updated October 9, 2020, ods.od.nih.gov/factsheets/VitaminD-HealthProfessional/.

238 600 to 800 IU per day: Harvard Women's Health Watch, "Taking Too Much Vitamin D Can Cloud Its Benefits and Create Health Risks," updated December 15, 2019, www.health.harvard.edu/staying-healthy/taking-too -much-vitamin-d-can-cloud-its-benefits-and-create-health-risks.

238 10 percent of our calories: U.S. Department of Health and Human Services, "2015–2020 Dietary Guidelines," health.gov/our-work/food-nutrition /2015–2020-dietary-guidelines/guidelines/chapter-2/a-closer-look-at-current -intakes-and-recommended-shifts/.

238 under 6 percent: American Heart Association, "Saturated Fat," www. heart.org/en/healthy-living/healthy-eating/eat-smart/fats/saturated-fats.

239 choosing lean cuts of meat: Office of Disease Prevention and Health Promotion, "Cut Down on Saturated Fats," *2015–2020 Dietary Guidelines for Americans,* December 2016, https://health.gov/sites/default/files/2019-10 /DGA_Cut-Down-On-Saturated-Fats.pdf.

239 preventing daytime sleepiness: Yingting Cao, Anne W. Taylor, Xiaoqun Pan, et al., "Dinner fat intake and sleep duration and self-reported sleep parameters over five years: Findings from the Jiangsu Nutrition Study of Chinese adults." *Nutrition* 32, no. 9 (2016): 970–74.

240 lighter, less restorative sleep: Marie-Pierre St-Onge, Anja Mikic, and Cara E. Pietrolungo, "Effects of diet on sleep quality." *Advances in Nutrition* 7, no. 5 (2016): 938–49.

240 ultra-processed foods: Larissa Galastri Baraldi, Euridice Martinez Steele, Daniela Silva Canella, and Carlos Augusto Monteiro, "Consumption of ultra-processed foods and associated sociodemographic factors in the USA between 2007 and 2012: Evidence from a nationally representative cross-sectional study." *BMJ Open* 8, no. 3 (2018): e020574.

240 excellent source of fiber: FiberFacts.org, "Dietary Fiber on the Food La-

bel," August 26, 2016, www.fiberfacts.org/dietary-fiber-food-label/; U.S. Food and Drug Administration. "CFR—Code of Federal Regulations Title 21," April 1, 2020, www.accessdata.fda.gov/scripts/cdrh/cfdocs/cfcfr/cfrsearch .cfm?fr=101.54.

240 fiber goal: Mayo Clinic, "Dietary fiber: Essential for a healthy diet," January 6, 2021, www.mayoclinic.org/healthy-lifestyle/nutrition-and-healthy -eating/in-depth/fiber/art-20043983.

241 excessive salt intake: Tomohiro Matsuo, Yasuyoshi Miyata, and Hideki Sakai, "Daily salt intake is an independent risk factor for pollakiuria and nocturia." *International Journal of Urology* 24, no. 5 (2017): 384–89.

241 well over the top: CDC, "Sodium and the Dietary Guidelines," October 2017, www.cdc.gov/salt/pdfs/sodium_dietary_guidelines.pdf.

241 from the CDC: "Sodium and the Dietary Guidelines," October 2017, www.cdc.gov/salt/pdfs/sodium_dietary_guidelines.pdf.

241 the Mayo Clinic: Mayo Clinic, "Sodium: How to tame your salt habit," June 29, 2019, www.mayoclinic.org/healthy-lifestyle/nutrition-and-healthy -eating/in-depth/sodium/art-20045479.

241 and the FDA: FDA, "Sodium in Your Diet," April 20, 2020, https:// www.fda.gov/food/nutrition-education-resources-materials/sodium-your-diet.

243 Mediterranean diet on sleep: Marie-Pierre St-Onge and Faris M. Zu-raikat, "Reciprocal roles of sleep and diet in cardiovascular health: A review of recent evidence and a potential mechanism." *Current Atherosclerosis Reports* 21, no. 3 (2019): 11; Isabelle Jaussent, Yves Dauvilliers, Marie-Laure Ancelin, et al., "Insomnia symptoms in older adults: Associated factors and gender differences." *American Journal of Geriatric Psychiatry* 19, no. 1 (2011): 88–97.

244 Harvard Health blog recommends: Katherine D. McManus, "A Practical Guide to the Mediterranean Diet," March 21, 2019, www.health.harvard .edu/blog/a-practical-guide-to-the-mediterranean-diet-2019032116194.

245 "option, not a necessity": W. Chris Winter, *The Sleep Solution: Why Your Sleep Is Broken and How to Fix It* (New York: New American Library, 2017), 121. Kindle.

246 isn't perfectly accurate: Vitor Teixeira, Silvia M. Voci, Raquel S. Mendes Netto, and Danielle G. da Silva, "The relative validity of a food record using the smartphone application MyFitnessPal." *Nutrition & Dietetics* 75, no. 2 (2018): 219–25.

Chapter 20: Relaxation Tools

252 achieving relaxation: Kenneth L. Lichstein, Daniel J. Taylor, Christina S. McCrae, S. Justin Thomas, chapter 4, "Relaxation for Insomnia," in Perelman School of Medicine, University of Pennsylvania, *BSM Treatment Protocols for Insomnia*, www.med.upenn.edu/cbti/assets/user-content/documents /Lichstein_RelaxationforInsomnia-BTSD.pdf.

252 not particularly stressed: Kenneth L. Lichstein, Daniel J. Taylor, Chris-tina S. McCrae, S. Justin Thomas, chapter 4, "Relaxation for Insomnia," in Perelman School of Medicine, University of Pennsylvania, *BSM Treatment*

Protocols for Insomnia, www.med.upenn.edu/cbti/assets/user-content/docu
ments/Lichstein_RelaxationforInsomnia-BTSD.pdf.

253 variants of relaxation: Kenneth L. Lichstein, Daniel J. Taylor, Christina S.
McCrae, S. Justin Thomas, chapter 4, "Relaxation for Insomnia," in Perelman
School of Medicine, University of Pennsylvania, *BSM Treatment Protocols
for Insomnia*, www.med.upenn.edu/cbti/assets/user-content/documents
/Lichstein_RelaxationforInsomnia-BTSD.pdf.

Chapter 22: Let There Be Dark

274 there's too much light: W. Chris Winter, *The Sleep Solution: Why Your
Sleep Is Broken and How to Fix It* (New York: New American Library, 2017),
108. Kindle.

275 activate the blue light sensors: Satchin Panda. *The Circadian Code: Lose
Weight, Supercharge Your Energy, and Transform Your Health from Morning to
Midnight* (New York: Rodale Books, 2018), 161–62. Kindle.

Chapter 23: Room/Bed Temperature

279 warm to cool is the mantra: Nick Littlehales, *Sleep: The Myth of 8 Hours,
the Power of Naps, and the New Plan to Recharge Your Body and Mind* (New
York: Da Capo Lifelong Books, 2017), 102. Kindle.

280 how quickly we'll fall asleep: Kurt Kräuchi, Christian Cajochen, Esther
Werth, and Anna Wirz-Justice, "Functional link between distal vasodila-
tion and sleep-onset latency?" *American Journal of Physiology—Regulatory,
Integrative and Comparative Physiology* 278, no. 3 (2000): R741–R748; Kurt
Kräuchi, Christian Cajochen, Esther Werth, and Anna Wirz-Justice, "Warm
feet promote the rapid onset of sleep." *Nature* 401, no. 6748 (1999): 36–37.

280 abnormally regulated skin temperature: Rolf Fronczek, Sebastiaan
Overeem, Gert Jan Lammers, J. Gert van Dijk, et al., "Altered skin-
temperature regulation in narcolepsy relates to sleep propensity." *Sleep* 29,
no. 11 (2006): 1444–49.

280 more sleep loss: Lynn Celmer, "Sleep deprivation disrupts regulation of
body heat," Sleep Education, December 18, 2012, sleepeducation.org/news
/2012/12/18/sleep-deprivation-disrupts-regulation-of-body-heat.

280 less than 12 minutes: Chika Oshima-Saeki, Yuiko Taniho, Hiromi Arita,
and Etsuko Fujimoto, "Lower-limb warming improves sleep quality in elderly
people living in nursing homes." *Sleep Science* 10, no. 2 (2017): 87–91.

280 an average 32 minutes: Yelin Ko and Joo-Young Lee, "Effects of feet
warming using bed socks on sleep quality and thermoregulatory responses in a
cool environment." *Journal of Physiological Anthropology* 37, no. 1 (2018): 1–11.

280 insulated slippers before bed: National Sleep Foundation, "Wearing
Socks to Bed: Is It Normal?" www.sleep.org/articles/wearing-socks-to-bed/.

284 "time to shut down": Arianna Huffington, *The Sleep Revolution: Transforming Your Life, One Night at a Time* (New York: Harmony Books, 2017), 223.
Kindle.

Chapter 24: Noise

287 a 2012 study: Kenneth I. Hume, Mark Brink, and Mathias Basner, "Effects of environmental noise on sleep." *Noise and Health* 14, no. 61 (2012): 297, https://www.noiseandhealth.org/article.asp?issn=1463-1741;year=2012;volume=14;issue=61;spage=297;epage=302;aulast=Hu.

289 "into healthy sleepers": Information in this interview is also supported by Gaelen Thomas Dickson and Emery Schubert, "Music on prescription to aid sleep quality: A literature review." *Frontiers in Psychology* 11 (2020): 1695; Gaelen Thomas Dickson and Emery Schubert, "How does music aid sleep? Literature review." *Sleep Medicine* 63 (2019): 142–50; Gaelen Thomas Dickson and Emery Schubert, "Musical features that aid sleep." *Musicae Scientiae* (2020): 1029864920972161.

Chapter 25: Snoring/Sleep Apnea Solutions

295 don't have sleep apnea: Christian Guilleminault, Riccardo Stoohs, and Stephen Duncan, "Snoring (I): daytime sleepiness in regular heavy snorers." *Chest* 99, no. 1 (1991): 40–48; Daniel J. Gottlieb, Qing Yao, Susan Redline, et al., "Does snoring predict sleepiness independently of apnea and hypopnea frequency?" *American Journal of Respiratory and Critical Care Medicine* 162, no. 4, pt 1 (2000): 1512–17.

303 impact is "limited": Cintia Zappe Fiori, Denis Martinez, Carolina Caruccio Montanari, et al., "Diuretic or sodium-restricted diet for obstructive sleep apnea—a randomized trial." *Sleep* 41, no. 4 (2018): zsy016.

Chapter 26: Mattress/Pillow

310 "time for a replacement": Jason Ellis, *The One-Week Insomnia Cure: Learn to Solve Your Sleep Problems* (London: Ebury Publishing, 2017), unpaginated. Kindle.

Chapter 27: Sharing

315 pediatric sleep experts: The Sleep Council (UK), "Sleep Advice for Children," sleepcouncil.org.uk/advice-support/sleep-advice/common-sleep-scenarios/sleep-advice-for-children/.

317 cuddle time: Jason Ellis, *The One-Week Insomnia Cure: Learn to Solve Your Sleep Problems* (London: Ebury Publishing, 2017), unpaginated. Kindle.

319 choosing sheets: The National Sleep Foundation, www.sleep.org/choosing-sheets.

320 or on the couch: "Adult Sleep Habits and Styles," Sleep Foundation, https://www.sleepfoundation.org/wp-content/uploads/2018/10/2005_summary_of_findings.pdf.

INDEX

ABC News, 2, 25, 64, 166, 175, 177, 184, 262–63, 317, 323
acid reflux, 154, 225, 301–302
  alcohol and, 301
  author's experience of, 2, 166, 227
  avoiding late meals, 151, 155–56, 227–28
  bed wedges for, 299
  sleep position for, 298
active cooling/heating systems, 285–86
acupuncturists, 207–208
acute insomnia, 43–45
Adaptive Servo-Ventilation (ASV), 22
adenoids, 19
adenosine, 85–86
  alcohol and, 198
  caffeine and, 215–16
ADHD (attention deficit hyperactivity disorder), 19
adjustable LEDs, 134
advanced body temperature rhythm, 146, 147–48
African Americans and sleep apnea, 17–18
Afrin (oxymetazoline nasal spray), 297
age, as predisposing factors, 42, 115
air travel. See also jet lag
  melatonin for, 142
  traveling east to west, 123, *123*, 132
  traveling west to east, 123, *123*, 132
alarm, last-call, 261–61
Alaska Sleep Clinic, 18, 225, 235
alcohol, 197–203, 257
  avoiding one hour before bedtime, 199–200
  avoiding sleep medications, 202
  body temperature and, 152
  core body temperature and, 146
  food and, 200–201
  hydration and, 201

"in moderation," 203
insomnia and, 50
prepping sleep environment before drinking, 201–202
snoring and, 301
taking breaks from, 202
withdrawal and insomnia, 28–29
allergies, 302–303
Amazon Echo, 289
Ambien
  author's use of, 2, 3–4, 68, 77
  Kendis Gibson's use of, 117
  Whit Johnson's use of, 46–47
ambient noise, 288–92
  colored noise, 290–91
  fans, 291–92
  music for, 288–89
  nature sounds, 291
Amdur, Adam, 15–16, 20
American Academy of Sleep Medicine (AASM), 39, 183, 192
American Osteopathic Association, 20–21
American Sleep Apnea Association, 15
America This Morning, 2, 62, 174
antibiotics, 19–20
antidepressants, 194
anti-distraction apps, 210
anxiety, 18, 55, 230
apartment dwellers, daytime sleep and doormen, 183
apnea. See sleep apnea
appetite, 48, 153–54
apps
  anti-distraction, 210
  BedTyme, 53–54
  CBT-i Coach, 30, 53, 100
  Entrain, 132
  food diaries, 245–46
  Shift Work App, 132, 176
  sleep diaries, 30

apps (*cont.*)
  Sleep On Cue, 35, 79–80, 94–95
  SnoreLab, 33, 34, 296
  Timeshifter, 132
Argonne diet, 159–60
  how-to, 159–60
Argonne National Laboratory, 159
armodafinil, 193–94
arousal, 55–57, *56*, 78, 201. *See also*
  conditioned arousal
arthritis, 166
astronauts, bright light therapy for, 129
attitude, 324–26
Audiobook/Podcast Test, 81–83
  how-to, 82
audio recordings, 34, 38
  snoring, 33, 34, 296
Ault, Trevor, 64–65, 177–78, 248, 289
auto accidents, 25, 181
autogenic training, 253
auto sleep recovery, 169
awake time, enjoyment of, 74–75

babies and sleep, 85, 115
baby monitors, 33
Babysleep.com, 39
back sleep position, 298, *306*, 306–307,
  309
baths, 148–49, 303
beans, 232, 239, 240, 244
bed bridges, 311
bedding (bedsheets), 281–83
BedJet, 285
bedroom environment. *See* sleep
  environment
bedroom zones, 314–15
beds. *See also* mattresses; pillows
  separate for partners (sleep divorce),
    320–22
"bed socks," 280–82
bed temperature, 277–78, 284–86
  chiliPAD for, 277–78, 283, 286
  right bedding, 281–83
bedtime
  early, 90–91, 168
  threat of wakefulness, 63–65

bedtime routine, 257–63
  avoiding overthinking, 263
  getting back on track (bedtime
    backtrack), 259
  lack of perfect formula, 259–60
  last-call alarm, 261–61
  routine vs. rigidity, 260–61
bedtime thoughts. *See* overactive mind
BedTyme, 53–54
bed wedges, 299
bedwetting and sleep apnea, 21
beer. *See* alcohol
Beth Israel Deaconess Medical Center,
  158
beverages, sleep-friendly, 244, 245
  herbal teas, 73, 157, 245
  tart cherry juice, 227, 245
Birmingham Behavioral Sleep Medicine
  Clinic, 39–40, 100
birth control pills and caffeine, 218
blackout coverings, 136–37, 272–74,
  293
  for doors, 273–74
  hand tests, 274–75
  measurements, 273
  portable blackout shades, 270–72
  side channels or panels, 273
  terminology, 272
  use of electrical tape, 274
  wraparound rods for, 272–73
blackout curtains, 268–69
blankets, 283–84, 316
bloating, 146
blood pressure, 15, 37, 165, 241, 287
blood sugar, 187, 234
blue light from screens, 125, 133,
  205–206
  blocking software, 212
BlueSleep Snoring, 18, 54
body temperature, 145–52, 278
  alcohol and, 152
  avoiding late, large meals, 151
  bright light therapy for, 147–48
  exercise timing and, 149–51
  melatonin and, 152
  sleep environment and, 151

warm hands and feet, 149, 279–81
warm showers/baths for, 148–49
body temperature rhythm, 146–48, 281
advanced, 146, 147–48
delayed, 145
bone health and vitamin D, 236
booze. *See* alcohol
boredom, 64–65
box springs, 309
Brad (author's friend), 32, 42, 65, 74–75, 97–98
brain dump, 69
breakfast, 153, 187
breastfeeding, 141
breathing rhythm, 248
breath work meditation, 76, 253–54
how-to, 253–54
Breus, Michael, 110, 167–68, 202, 216, 217, 222
bright light therapy, 128–33
body temperature and, 147–48
how-to, 130–32, 179
keeping it comfortable and convenient, 133
light timing calculator, 132
brightness adjustments on screens, 211–12
Brown, Timothy, 134
Burgess, Helen, 140–41, 142, 143, 168, 179
"burning calories," 149–50
butter, 239

caffeine (coffee), 157, 215–24, 326–27
air travel and, 160
avoiding before bedtime, 217–19
avoiding stimulants with, 223
Brad's experience, 32
caffeine and, 215–17
circadian effects of, 218–19
cognitive performance and, 180
functions of, 215–16
graveyard shift workers and, 171–72, 180
napping and, 220–21
phase delay of, 224

ritual morning, moving to later, 215–17
routine reset, 221–22
schedule, 215–17
sleep inertia vs., 220–21 216
tapering techniques, 222–23
tolerance of, 217, 221–22
Whit Johnson's experience, 46
worrying about, 224
calorie counting, 245–46
cannabis, 28–29
car accidents, 25, 181
carbohydrates, 154, 188, 200, 226
fiber and, 240
in Mediterranean diet, 243
tryptophan and, 233–34
whole grains, 232, 234, 240, 244
car sleeping, 85
cataplexy, 25
causation vs. correlation, 48
CBS New York, 2–3, 175, 323
CBT-I. *See* cognitive behavioral therapy for insomnia
CBT-i Coach, 30, 53, 100
central sleep apnea, 16
Cervo Brain Research Centre, 189
children and sleep apnea, 19–21
Marco's story, 19–20
symptoms, 20–21
ChiliPAD, 277–78, 283, 286
chin straps, 300
chronic insomnia, 43–45, 51, *92*
diet's role in, 226
elevated cortisol levels and, 154, 226, 234
intensive sleep retraining for, 93–96
chronotype questionnaire, 112
how-to, 113
chronotypes, 109–13
early birds/morning type. *See* early birds
graveyard shift workers and, 173–74
hummingbirds/intermediate type, 110, *110*
night owls/evening type. *See* night owls
scheduling, 115–23

cigarettes. *See* smoking
Circadian Code, The (Panda), 126, 128,
    154, 155, 156–57, 161, 223, 275
circadian rhythm, 4, 10, *10*, 105–107
    author's experience, 107
    caffeine's effects, 218–19
    chronotypes, 109–13
    consistent wake-up time and, 122,
        165
    exercise to advance, 161–62
    exercise to delay, 162–63
    five hours ahead sleep schedule, 118,
        118
    five hours behind sleep schedule, 117,
        117
    graveyard shift workers and, 171–72
    light/dark contrast, 125–37
    meal timing and, 153
    schedules, 105–106, *106*, 115–23
circadian rhythm disorders
    diagnosis of, 13–14
    diet's role, 226
circadian shifting
    compromise circadian position,
        178–80
    for graveyard shift workers, 176
    melatonin for, 140–42
circulatory issues, 147, 152, 280
classical conditioning, 60, 252, 257
clockwise rotations, 123, 192
coffee. *See* caffeine
cognitive behavioral therapy for
        insomnia (CBT-I), 51–54
    BedTyme, 53–54
    CBT-i Coach, 30, 53, 100
    digital, 52
    sleep compression, 100–104
    Sleepio, 52–53
    sleep restriction, 97–100
    Somryst, 52
    stimulus control, 96–97, 102
cognitive performance and coffee, 180
colored noise, 290–91
Color Filters settings, 209
color temperature, 133–34
color tone of screens, 133–34, 212

Columbia University Irving Medical
    Center's Sleep Center of
    Excellence, 229
compromise circadian position, 178–80
    how-to, 180
conditioned arousal, 6, 60–61, 63, 87,
    249, 327
    author's experience, 61, 66, 107
    cortisol and, 154, 226
Consensus Sleep Diary, 30–31, 189
    how-to DIY, 31
consistency
    in schedule, 102, 174–76
    in wake time, 122, 165
constructive worry, 45, 68–71, 74, 224,
    250
    adjustments, 70–71
    how-to, 70
Cook, Tim, 115
corneal disease, 49–50
correlation vs. causation, 48
cortisol, 226, 230, 234
    caffeine and, 216
    carbohydrates and, 154
    chronic insomnia and elevated, 154,
        226, 234
    circadian rhythm and, 125, 145
    Jason Karp's experience, 49, 63
Covid-19 pandemic, 5, 183, 208, 302
CPAP (continuous positive airway
    pressure), 14–15, 16, 21–22, 304
Cramps, 146
Cure for Jet Lag, The (Ehret), 159
cytochrome inhibitors, 218

dark chocolate, 223
darkness fixes, 125–28
    bright light therapy, 128–33
    Four D's (dimness, distance,
        duration, direction), 126–28
dark sleep environment, 267–76. *See
    also* blackout coverings
    blackout curtains, 268–69
    eyelids and light sensitivity, 267–68
    mood lighting, 276
    motion sensor strip lighting, 275, 318

portable blackout shades, 270–72
  sleep masks, 269–70
daytime sleepers. *See* graveyard shift
  workers
daytime sunlight, light exposure chart,
  135, *135*
delayed body temperature rhythm, 145
dementia, 15, 141
dental hygiene, 47, 196
dental problems, 166
depression, 18, 23, 28, 194, 233, 235
diabetes, 15, 141, 165
diagnosis, 11–40, 188
  asking your partner to help, 32–33
  audio recordings for, 34
  circadian rhythm disorders, 13–14
  finding right sleep specialists, 38–40
  Gotcha Alarm, 38
  insomnia, 12–13
  mental health issues, 27–28
  misdiagnosis, 11–12
  narcolepsy, 25–27
  parasomnias, 24–25
  periodic limb movement disorder, 24
  questionnaires, 36–37
  restless legs syndrome, 22–24
  sleep apnea/sleep disordered
    breathing, 14–22
  sleep diaries for, 29–32
  Spoon Test, 35–36
  substances and withdrawal insomnia,
    28–29
  video recordings for, 33–34
diaries. *See also* journaling; sleep diaries
  food diary apps, 245–46
diarrhea, 232
Dickson, Thomas, 288–92
diet, 225–46. *See also* meal timing;
  sleep nutrition; time-restricted
  eating
  alcohol and, 200–201
  author's experience, 225, 227–28
  avoiding late, large meals, 151,
    155–56
  body temperature and, 146, 151
  food diary apps, 245–46

graveyard shift workers and meal
    plans, 186–88
  insomnia and, 50
  Mediterranean, 243–44
  pre-bed snacks, 155–56, 226, 227–28
  sleep debt compared with, 166
dietary fats, 238–39
dietary fiber, 223, 240, 243
Dietary Guidelines for Americans, 229,
    238
  alcohol intake, 203
  saturated fats, 239
  sodium intake, 241
difference makers, 326–27
digital CBT-I, 52
digital sleep restriction, 100
dim/dark mode on screens, 211–12
dimming lights, 127–28
dimness, 126–28
dogs, sharing bed with, 319
doing less, 73–74
"Do Not Disturb" phone setting,
    182–83, 292–93
door blackout, 273–74
Drake, Christopher, 218
DriftTV, 212
drinking. *See* alcohol
drinking water, 156, 158, 201
drinks, sleep-friendly, 244, 245
  herbal teas, 73, 157, 245
  tart cherry juice, 227, 245
*Dropping Acid: The Reflux Diet
    Cookbook & Cure* (Stern), 302
drug substances and withdrawal
    insomnia, 28–29
dry eyes, 166
Duke University School of Medicine, 83
Dumaplin, Cara, 85–86

ear infections, and sleep apnea, 19–20
early bedtime, 90–91, 168
early birds (early risers), *109*, 109–10
  exercise schedule for, 162
  going to bed with partner at different
    times, 317
  schedules, 115–23, 174

earplugs, 270, 288
eating. *See* diet; time-restricted eating
Ehret, Charles, 159
eight-hours sleep myth, 3, 43, 87–89
   orthosomnia and, 88–89
Eight Sleep Pod, 285
elderly, 129, 147, 152
electrolytes, 201
Elliot, Janine, 174, 175, 178, 187
Elliott, David, meditations, 254
Ellis, Jason, 24–25, 38, 44, 64, 83, 97,
   310, 317
environment. *See* sleep environment
Erichsen, Daniel, 53, 66
   relaxation techniques, 250–51, 255
   sleep compression, 100–101
   sleep restriction, 98
ethnic minorities and sleep apnea,
   17–18
evening types. *See* night owls
exercise, 104, 161–63
   to advance circadian rhythm, 161–62
   building up sleep drive, 178
   to delay circadian rhythm, 162–63
   for RLS, 23
   timing and body temperature,
   149–51
eyelids and light sensitivity, 267–68

fans, 291–92
fasting, 154, 225. *See also* time-
   restricted eating
   for jet lag/shift work, 157–58
fatigue, 18, 91–93
   signs of, 91
fats, 238–39
Ferriss, Tim, 277–78
fiber, 223, 240, 243
fight-or-flight response, 64
Figueiro, Mariana, 129, 133, 148,
   267–68
fish, 236, 238, 239, 244
floor tests for mattresses, 308
foam mattresses, 311–12
food diary apps, 245–46
food labels, 240, 242

foot warming, 149, 280–81
forgetfulness, 62
Forgetting Sarah Marshall (movie), 325
45-minute sleep-in, 167–68
Four D's (dimness, distance, duration,
   direction), 126–28
Fox Business Network, 2, 323
Freeman, Kevin, 166

GABA (gamma aminobutyric acid), 230
gel pads, 285
genetics, as predisposing factors, 42,
   115
Gibson, Kendis, 117–18, 185
glasses. *See also* sunglasses
   for allergies, 302
   blue-light blocking, 137, 212
gluten, 50, 240
Good Morning America (GMA), 2, 5,
   38, 54, 62, 88, 174–75
Gotcha Alarm, 38
Grandner, Michael, 167, 261, 327
   relaxation tools, 248, 253, 257
   screens, 205–206, 208, 209
gratitude journals, 73
graveyard shift workers, 171–94
   author's experience, 1–4, 62–63,
     174–75, 181, 182–83, 185–86, 187
   building up sleep drive, 177–78
   caffeine and, 171–72, 180
   chronotype considerations, 173–74
   circadian shifting for, 176
   clockwise rotations for, 123, 192
   compromise circadian position,
     178–80
   enlisting sleep support, 184–86
   exercise for, 162–63
   fasting for, 157–58
   importance of consistency, 174–76
   light timing calculator, 132
   meal planning, 186–88
   modafinil for, 193–94
   napping for, 177–78, 180–82
   protecting your sleep, 182–83
   role of undiagnosed sleep disorders,
     188

Shift Work App, 132, 176
sleep diary, 189, *190*
sleeping pills for, 191–92
sleep time, not free time, 173
stimulus control, 190–91
sun block for, 136–37
weekend considerations, 177–79
gray noise, 290–91
grayscale trick for screens, 208–209
Greenburg, Jonathan, 22
green leafy vegetables, 232, 244
Grymes, Andrea, 175, 187
gut microbiome, 243

habits. *See* sleep habits
hair loss, 166
hand tests, 274–75
Harris, Dan, 68, 88–89, 231, 251–52, 320, 321
Harvard Medical School, 13, 36, 132, 158, 238
headaches, 14, 18, 21, 46–47, 47, 146, 222
headphone headband, 292
healthy snacks, 155–56, 187, 227
heartburn, 3, 225
heart conditions, 15, 16
heart rate, 64
Henry Ford Health System, 198–99, 218
herbal teas, 73, 157, 245
high blood pressure (hypertension), 15, 37, 241, 287
high core body temperature, 145–46
Hispanic Americans and sleep apnea, 17–18
home sleep studies, 21
Huffington, Arianna, 3, 86, 284
hummingbirds, 110, *110*
hunger, 85, 154
hydration (drinking water), 156, 158, 201

identifying the problem. *See* diagnosis
indigestion, 153–54
innerspring mattresses, 311–12

insomnia, 41–54
author's mother's experience of, 41–42, 44
CBT-I for, 51–54
circadian rhythm disorders compared with, 13–14
definition of, 12, 13, 43, 48
depression and, 28
diagnosis, 12–13
diet's role, 225–26
doctors and sleeping pills, 46–47
insomniac vs. person with, 45
Jason Karp's experience of, 48–50
"just how you are," 41–42
not sleepy enough, 85–104
overactive mind. *See* overactive mind
parasomnia compared with, 24–25
prevalence of, 41
RLS compared with, 23
schedules, 119–20
self-help alternatives, 54
sleep apnea and, 17
"sleep debt doom" narrative, 48–50
sleep deprivation vs., 43
truth about sleep hygiene, 47
types of, 43–45
visiting your doctor, 51
Whit Johnson's experience of, 38, 46–47
insomniac (term), 45
insulin, 153, 158, 234
insulin resistance, 165
intensive sleep retraining (ISR), 93–96
how-to, 95–96
interruptions
enlisting sleep support, 184–86
protecting your sleep, 182–83, 292–93
iPhones. *See* apps; smartphones
iron deficiency and RLS, 23

jaw clenching, 21
jet lag
Argonne diet for, 159–60
fasting for, 157–58
light timing for, 130, 131–32

jet lag (*cont.*)
  melatonin for, 142
  social. *See* social jet lag
  traveling east to west, 123, *123*, 132
  traveling west to east, 123, *123*, 132
Johns Hopkins University School of
  Medicine, 28, 149–50
Johnson, Dwayne "the Rock," 115
Johnson, Whit, 38, 46–47, 248
journaling (journals), 72–73
  gratitude, 73
  how-to, 72
*Journal of the American Osteopathic
  Association*, 19

Kane, Eliza, 253–54
Karp, Jason, 48–50, 63, 69, 75, 86, 104,
  166
Kingston, Kofi, 104, 116, 121
Kleitman, Nathaniel, 35
Kondo, Marie, 71
Krakow, Barry, 22

last-call alarm, 261–61
late (terminal) insomnia, 43
layers of coverings, 282–83
legumes, 240, 244
light/dark contrast, 125–37
  bright light therapy, 128–33
  Four D's (dimness, distance,
    duration, direction), 126–28
  light exposure chart, 135, *135*
  lighting color/tone, 133–34
  screen hacks, 136
  sun block, 136–37
light fixes. *See* blackout coverings;
    bright light therapy; dark sleep
    environment
lighting
  adjustable LEDs, 134
  color/tone, 133–34
  dimming lights, 127–28
  eyelids and light sensitivity, 267–68
  graveyard shift workers and, 136–37
  lamps, 127
  light exposure chart, 135, *135*

mood, 276
  night-lights, 128, 134
  use of electrical tape, 274
light sensitivity and eyelids, 267–68
light therapy. *See* bright light therapy
light-tight sleep environment. *See* dark
  sleep environment
light timing calculator, 132
line test for mattresses, *306*, 306–307,
  310
  how-to, 306–307
Littlehales, Nick, 279, 309–10, 316
liver and alcohol intake, 200–201
liver disease, 15, 217–18
Lockley, Steven, 13, 132
low body temperature, 146–47
Ludwig-Maximilian University, 112
Lux, 126–27, 129, 136
  light exposure chart, 135, *135*

magnesium, 230–32
  food sources of, 232
  for PLMD, 24, 231
  recommended daily allowance
    (RDA), 231, *231*
  for RLS, 23, 231
  testing for deficiency, 231–32
  toxicity, 232
malted milk, 226
marijuana, 28–29
Matrix, The (movie), 67
mattresses, 305–12
  adding firmness, 309
  adding softness, 308
  chiliPAD for, 277–78, 283, 286
  floor tests for, 308
  insulation level of, 311–12
  line test for, 306–307, 310
  pressure points, 307–308
  return policy, 312
  right bedding for, 281–83
  size of, 310–11, 316
  temperature control, 284–86,
    311–12
mattress toppers, 308
Mayo Clinic, 15, 54, 240

meal timing, 153–60. *See also* time-restricted eating
  Argonne diet, 159–60
  fasting for jet lag/shift work, 157–58
  midnight snacks, 153, 155–56, 227–28
medications. *See* sleeping pills
meditation, 76, 248, 249, 251–54. *See also* breath work meditation
  author's experience, 66–68, 247, 248, 251
  myth of the "quiet mind," 66–68
Mediterranean diet, 243–44
  how-to, 244
Medley, Dorinda, 326
melatonin
  body temperature and, 152
  darkness and circadian rhythm, 125, 126–27, 136
  right way to take, 139–43
  for sleep onset, 143
melatonin for circadian shifting, 140–42
  how-to, 141–42
melatonin timing, 132
memory and overactive mind, 62
menopause, 19, 146
  sleep apnea and, 19
menstruation, 146
mental breaks, 62–63, 75
mental health issues, diagnosis of, 27–28
metabolic syndrome, 15
metabolism, 42, 200
midnight snacks, 151, 153, 155–56, 226, 227–28
mindfulness, 249, 251, 253
  author's experience, 66–68
  myth of the "quiet mind," 66–68
minorities and sleep apnea, 17–18
mobile phones. *See* screens; smartphones
modafinil, 193–94
mood, 15, 178, 194, 233, 235
mood lighting, 276
morning types. *See* early birds

motion sensor strip lighting, 275, 318
mount tape, 300
mouth guards, 299–300
Mundt, Jennifer, 259, 260
Munich Chronotype Questionnaire (MCTQ), 112–13
muscle relaxers, 301
music, for sound masking, 288–89
Musk, Elon, 120
myths. *See* sleep myths

naps (napping), 89–90, *90*, 168–69
  building up sleep drive, 177–78
  caffeine and, 220–21
  for graveyard shift workers, 177–78, 180–82
narcolepsy
  diagnosis of, 25–27
  Ginger Zee's experience, 25–27
nasal rinses, 303
nasal spray, 297
nasal strips, 270, 296–97
National Institutes of Health, 141, 236, 237
National Sleep Foundation, 23, 87, 104, 168, 169, 221, 230, 234, 277, 280, 282, 320
Native Americans and sleep apnea, 17–18
nature sounds, 291
Netflix, autoplay feature, 210
nicotine. *See also* smoking
  withdrawal insomnia and, 28–29
night-lights, 128
  red, 134
nightmares, 26
night owls (evening types), 111, *111*, 263
  exercise schedule for, 162
  going to bed with partner at different times, 317
  graveyard shift workers and, 173–74
  schedules, 115, 116–17, 120–21, 137, 173–74
night shift workers. *See* graveyard shift workers

nighttime light exposure chart, 135,
    135
nighttime snacks, 151, 153, 155–56,
    226, 227–28
noise, 287–93
    "Do Not Disturb," 182–83, 292–93
    earplugs, 270, 288
    headphone headband, 292
    partner sights/sounds, 317–19
    sound masking, 288–92
Nooyi, Indra, 115
Northumbria Centre for Sleep
    Research, 24–25, 44
Northwestern Memorial Hospital
    Center for Circadian & Sleep
    Medicine, 65
Northwestern University Feinberg
    School of Medicine, 259
nose cones, 297
notebooks, 71. *See also* sleep diaries
    constructive worry lists, 70–71
    journaling, 72–73
nutritional supplements. *See also* sleep
    nutrition
    warning, 230
nutrition labels, 240, 242
nuts, 232, 239, 240, 244

obstructive sleep apnea, 16–17
Ohanian, Alexis, 120
olive oil, 239, 244
O'Neal, Shaquille, 21–22
O'Neill, John, 153–54, 158, 219
One-Week Insomnia Cure, The (Ellis),
    64, 310
Ong, Jason, 32, 65, 119–20, 122, 224,
    249
open windows, 303
oral contraceptives and caffeine, 218
orthodontic expanders, 19
orthosomnia, 88–89
Oura Ring, 88
overactive mind, 59–76
    author's routine for, 60
    carrying on, 76
    conditioned arousal, 60–61

constructive worry, 68–71
    doing less, 73–74
    enjoying awake time, 74–75
    journaling, 72–73
    memory, 62
    mental downtime, 62–63
    "quiet mind" myth, 66–68
    relaxation tools. *See* relaxation tools
        and techniques
    "sleep through the night" myth,
        65–66
    threat of wakefulness, 63–65
overnight workers. *See* graveyard shift
    workers
oxymetazoline nasal spray (Afrin),
    297

pajamas, 283–84
Panda, Satchin
    diet, 151, 154, 155, 156–57
    exercise, 161
    lighting, 126, 128, 134, 275
    stimulants, 223
Panfel, Sandy, 315–16
parasomnias, diagnosis of, 24–25
partners
    diagnosis from, 32–33
    enlisting sleep support, 184–86
    sharing. *See* sharing
passive attitude, 251–52, 324–26
peanut butter, 188, 227
periodic limb movement disorder
    (PLMD), 24
    magnesium for, 24, 231
personal bedding, 282
pets, sharing bed with, 319
phone screens. *See* screens
Pierpaoli Parker, Christina, 39–40
Pilgrim, Eva, 146, 147, 269, 273, 286
pillows, 283, 309–10
    wedge, 299
pink noise, 290–91
placebo effect, 232
podcasts, 62, 64, 191
Podcast Test, 81–83
    how-to, 82

pollen protection, 302–303
Portable blackout shades, 270–72
    how-to DIY, 271
Posner, Donn, 88
Power of When, The (Breus), 167–68
pre-bed snacks, 155–56, 226, 227–28
pregnancy, 19, 141, 218, 310
pressure points, 307–308
progressive muscle relaxation, 253

questionnaires, 36–37
    chronotypes, 112–13
    STOP-Bang, 37
"quiet mind" myth, 66–68

racial minorities and sleep apnea,
    17–18
Railroaders' Guide to Healthy Sleep,
    189
Raymann, Roy
    body temperature, 146–47, 148
    mattresses, 310–12, 316
    room/bed temperature, 279, 280,
        281–82, 285
reading, 74–75
red night-lights, 134
relaxation tools and techniques, 76,
    247–55
    appreciating the exercise, 250–51
    constructive worry, 250
    experimenting with, 253–54
    passive attitude, 251–52
    practicing daily, 252
relaxed attitude, 251–52, 324–26
REM (rapid eye movement) sleep,
    65–66, 169, 233
restless legs syndrome (RLS), 22–24,
    198
    author's mother's experience, 23
    diagnosis of, 22–23
    magnesium for, 23, 231
    treatment of, 23–24
reverse curfew, 103–104
RLS. *See* restless legs syndrome
Roehrs, Timothy, 198–200, 201
Roenneberg, Till, 112

room temperature, 277–86
    pajamas, 283–84
    right bedding, 281–83
    warm hands and feet, 149, 279–81
    warm to cool, 279
Rosa (author's cousin), 19–20
Rosemary (author's friend), 283
rotating fixes, 123, 192
rotating shift workers, 123, *123*
Rush University, 207
Rutgers Medical School Division of
    Sleep and Circadian Medicine,
    129

St-Onge, Marie-Pierre, 200, 229–30,
    238, 240, 243, 245
Salk Institute for Biological Studies,
    134
salt. *See* sodium
Saper, Clifford, 158
saturated fats, 238–39
    how-to cut down on, 238–39
    timing, 239
scheduling (schedules), 115–23
    chronotype considerations, 120–21
    circadian rhythm vs., 105–106, *106*
    exercise, 149–51, 161–63
    five hours ahead sleep schedule, 118,
        118
    five hours behind sleep schedule, 117,
        117
    for insomnia, 119–20
    moving east to west, 123, *123*
    shift workers in disguise, 116–19
    social jet lag, 119
Schur, Carolyn, 121, 174, 184–85,
    187–88
Scott, Hannah, 93–95
screens, 136, 205–13
    blue light from, 125, 133, 205–206,
        212
    brightness adjustments, 211–12
    bright side of, 207–208
    distance from, 213
    grayscale trick, 208–209
    lighting color/tone, 133–34, 212

screens (*cont.*)
  opting for passive activities, 210
  the rabbit hole, 205–207
  standing up while using, 209
  time curfew, 73, 182–83, 208, 210
seeds, 232, 239, 240, 244
seniors (elderly), 129, 147, 152
separate beds or bedrooms (sleep
    divorce), 320–22
serotonin, 233, 234, 235
sharing, 313–22
  going to bed at different times, 317
  partner sights/sounds, 317–19
  with pets, 319
  room zones, 314–15
Sheahan, Jack, 175–76
sheets, 281–83
shift work (workers), 116–19. *See also*
    graveyard shift workers
  fasting for, 158
  five hours ahead sleep schedule, 118,
    118
  five hours behind sleep schedule, 117,
    117
  light timing calculator, 132
  overnight exercise for, 162–63
Shift Work App, 132, 176
showers, 148–49, 303
side sleep position, 298, *306*, 306–307,
    309–10
skin cancer, 237
skin temperature. *See* body
    temperature
sleep apnea, 14–22
  assessment, 37
  audio recording, 34
  author's father's experience, 14–15,
    19, 22
  avoiding diagnosis, 21–22
  children and, 19–21
  diagnosis of, 14–17
  insomnia and, 17
  minorities and, 17–18
  risks, 15
  solutions for snoring, 295–304.
    See also snoring

symptoms, 16, 18
  women and, 18–19
Sleep Apnea Center, 18
sleep compression, 100–104
  author's experience, 102–103
  how-to, 101
sleep confidence, 77–78, 199, 327
sleep debt, 165–67
"sleep debt doom," 48–50
sleep debt strategies, 167–69
  auto sleep recovery, 169
  earlier bedtime, 168
  fixing sleep disorders first, 167
  45-minute sleep-in, 167–68
  napping, 168–69
sleep deprivation
  definition of, 43, 48
  insomnia vs., 43, 48
sleep diaries, 29–32, 74
  apps, 30
  for graveyard shift workers, 189,
    190
sleep disordered breathing, 14–22
  diagnosis of, 14–17
sleep divorce, 320–22
sleep drive, 9, *9*, 55–57, *56*, 78, *85*,
    85–86, 89
  circadian rhythm, 105–106, *106*
sleep environment, 47, 201–202
  body temperature and, 151
  darkness, 267–76
  mattresses/pillows, 305–12
  noise, 287–93
  overview of, 265
  room/bed temperature, 277–86
  sharing, 313–22
  snoring/sleep apnea solutions,
    295–304
Sleep Foundation, 17, 197
sleep habits, 47
  alcohol, 197–203
  bedtime routine, 257–63
  caffeine, 215–24
  diet, 225–28
  dos and don'ts, 195–96
  nutrition, 229–46

overview of, 195–96
partner and, 18
relaxation tools, 76, 247–55
screens, 205–13
sleep hygiene, 4, 47, 195–96. *See also*
    sleep environment; sleep habits
sleep inertia, 216
    caffeine vs., 220–21 216
    napping and, 181–82
sleepiness, 91–93
    questionnaire, 36
sleeping in, 89–90, *90*, 119
    45 minutes, 167–68
sleeping pills (medications). *See also*
    Ambien
    avoiding alcohol, 202
    doctors and insomnia, 46–47
    for parasomnia, 25
    for shift workers, 191–92
    tolerance of, 3–4
Sleepio, 52–53
sleep masks, 269–70, 318
sleep misperception, 77–84, *78*
    Audiobook/Podcast Test, 81–83
    Sleep On Cue, 35, 79–80, 94–95
    Tally Test, 83
    Tissue Test, 80–81
sleep music playlists, 289–90
sleep myths, 247–48
    eight-hours sleep, 3, 43, 87–89
    "quiet mind," 66–68
    sleep apnea and obesity, 18
    "sleep debt doom," 48–50
    "sleep through the night," 65–66
sleep nutrition, 229–46
    fats, 238–39
    fiber, 240
    magnesium, 230–32
    sodium, 241–42
    tryptophan, 233–34
    vitamin B6, 235–36
    vitamin D, 236–38
Sleep On Cue, 79–80, 94–95
    Custom Nap function, 35, 79
    how-to, 79–80
sleep paralysis, 25–26

sleep position, 298–99, *306*, 306–307,
    309–10
sleep problems, identifying. *See*
    diagnosis
sleep restriction, 97–100
    digital, 100
    how-to, 98–99
Sleep Revolution, The (Huffington), 3,
    86, 284
sleep schedule. *See* scheduling
SleepScore Labs, 147
sleep seesaw, 55–57, *56*, 78, *78*
Sleep Smarter (Stevenson), 223
Sleep Solution, The (Winter), 245,
    274–75
sleep specialists, 11
    finding, 38–40
    resources, 39
sleep studies, 39, 42, 304
    author's experience, 77–78
    at home, 21
"sleep suffocation." *See* sleep apnea
sleep support, enlisting, 184–86
sleepwalking, 24
sleep zones, 315–16
smartphones. *See also* apps; screens
    "Do Not Disturb" phone setting,
        182–83, 292–93
    grayscale trick for, 208–209
    standing up while using, 209
    Tally Test, 83
smoking
    caffeine and, 217–18
    core body temperature and, 146
    withdrawal insomnia and, 28–29
sniffing sleep position, 298–99, 309
SnoreLab, 33, 34, 296
snoring, 295–304
    allergies and, 302–303
    audio recordings of, 33, 34, 296
    avoiding drinking late at night and,
        301
    bed wedges for, 299
    chin straps/mount tape, 300
    mouth guards for, 299–300
    opening your nose, 296–97

snoring (*cont.*)
  partner and, 319
  sleep position and, 298–99
  SnoreLab app, 33, 34, 296
  sodium and, 303
  weight loss for, 301
snowball effect, 328
Sobel, Liz, 184
social jet lag, 119, 177
  compromise circadian position for, 179
  exercise schedule for, 162
Society of Behavioral Sleep Medicine, 39
sodium (salt), 241–42, 303
  how-to cut down on, 241–42
Somryst, 52
sound masking, 288–92
  colored noise, 290–91
  fans, 291–92
  music for, 288–89
  nature sounds, 291
spectrum fixes, 133–34, 212
speech delays and sleep apnea, 21
Spoon Test, 35–36, 80
  how-to, 35–36
Stern, Jordan, 18, 21, 34, 39, 54, 102, 295–303
Stevenson, Shawn, 223
stimulants, 223
stimulus control, 96–97, 102, 168
  how-to, 96–97
  for shift workers, 190–91
stomach sleep position, 298, *306*, 306–307, 309
stomach upset, 232
STOP-Bang Questionnaire, 37
  how-to, 37
stress, 165, 230, 249, 287
strokes, 15
substances and withdrawal insomnia, 28–29
sun block. *See* blackout coverings
sunglasses, 14, 128, 136–37, 213
  for allergies, 302
  blue-light blocking, 137, 212

sunlight and vitamin D, 237
sunscreen, 237
supplements. *See also* sleep nutrition
  warning, 230

Tally Test, 83
  how-to, 83
tart cherry juice, 227, 245
teeth grinding, 21, 24
temperature. *See* bed temperature; body temperature; room temperature
Ten Percent Happier (podcast), 88
10% Happier and Meditation for Fidgety Skeptics (Harris), 68
terminal insomnia, 43
THC (tetrahydrocannabinol), 28–29
thermoregulation, 146
THIM smart ring, 94–95
Thomas, Justin, 98, 100–101
thread count of sheets, 282
throat infections, and sleep apnea, 19–20
time-restricted eating (TRE), 154, 156–58, 228
  how-to, 156–57
  for jet lag/shift work, 157–58
Timeshifter, 132
  Shift Work App, 132, 176
timing meals. *See* meal timing
tiredness, 91–93
"tired tank," 85–86, 89
Tissue Test, 80–81
  how-to, 80–81
toe warmers, 280–81
Tom (author's husband), 24, 87, 89, 91, 94, 103, 127, 175, 184–85, 187, 207, 208, 260, 261, 262, 267, 268, 275, 277–78, 282–83, 309, 313–14, 317–18, 321, 322, 323–24, 330
tonsillectomies, 19, 20
Tools of Titans (Ferriss), 277–78
training effect, 150
Tran, Nga, 57
traveling east to west, 123, *123*, 132
  melatonin for, 142

traveling west to east, 123, *123*, 132
  melatonin for, 142
tryptophan, 233–34
TV watching, 74, 75, 250–51, 258, 259, 261, 262. *See also* screens
  changing color tone, 212
  distance from, 213
  opting for passive activities, 210
two-zoned mattresses, 310–11, 316
type 2 diabetes, 15

University of Arizona College of Medicine, 167
University of Chicago, 35, 165
University of Michigan, 132
University of Michigan Medical School's Sleep and Circadian Research Laboratory, 140

valerian tea, 245
Vallières, Annie, 189, 190–92
Vandrey, Ryan, 28–29
video recordings, 33–34, 38
  Tissue Test, 80–81
vitamin B₆, 235–36
  food sources of, 236
  recommended daily allowance (RDA), *235*, 235–36
vitamin D, 236–38
  food sources of, 238
  recommended daily allowance (RDA), 237, *237*
  from the sun, 237

Wahlberg, Mark, 115, 121
wakefulness, 63–65, 97
  body temperature and, 147–48
  modafinil for, 193–94
  threat of, 63–65
wake time, consistency in, 122, 165
waking up too early, 43, 89, 122, 127, 146
Walker, Matthew, 3, 139
warming hands or feet, 149, 279–81
warm showers/baths, 148–49
water, drinking, 156, 158, 201

wedge pillows, 283, 299
weekends and graveyard shift worker considerations, 177–79
weight gain, 154
weight loss, 243, 301
white noise, 290–91
whole grains, 232, 234, 240, 244
Why We Sleep (Walker), 3, 139
Wignall, Nick, 27–28, 68, 73, 328
Williams, Pharrell, 120–21
Willis-Ekbom disease. *See* restless legs syndrome
window coverings. *See* blackout coverings
wine, 199, 202, 244, 258. *See also* alcohol
Winter, Chris, 181, 245
  alcohol use, 202
  hand tests, 274–75
  mattresses, 307, 312
  modafinil, 193, 194
  stimulants, 223
women and sleep apnea, 18–19
working out. *See* exercise
work schedules
  employer considerations, 121
  five hours ahead sleep schedule, 118, *118*
  five hours behind sleep schedule, 117, *117*
  graveyard shifts. *See* graveyard shift workers
  light timing calculator, 132
  shift workers in disguise, 116–19
World News Now, 2, 5, 62, 174
wraparound rods for blackout coverings, 272–73
Wright, Ken, 219, 220, 221, 224
Wu, Jade, 81, 83, 260
Wyatt, James, 207, 217, 222–23

Young, Paul, 307, 308
Youngstedt, Shawn, 150, 162–63

Zee, Ginger, 25–27, 193–94
Zuckerberg, Mark, 120

ABOUT THE AUTHOR

Diane Macedo is an Emmy Award–winning journalist who is currently an anchor and correspondent for ABC News and ABC News Live. As a lifelong night owl who has worked virtually every schedule imaginable, Diane is the last person anyone ever expected to write about sleep. But she's also a *tiny* bit stubborn, life-hack obsessed, and incapable of leaving a puzzle unfinished. So it's no surprise that she set out to find answers to her insomnia and didn't stop until she'd written a book full of sleep solutions. When she's not chasing news or sleep fixes, Diane can be found singing, hiking, cooking, or otherwise enjoying family time—probably trying to do too many things at once.

You can catch her on Instagram, Twitter, and Facebook at @dianermacedo.